JEANNE S. RINGEL, JULIA LEJEUNE, JESSICA PHILLIPS, MICHAEL W. ROBBINS, MELISSA A. BRADLEY, JOSHUA WOLF, MARTHA J. TIMMER

Understanding Veterans in New York

A Needs Assessment of Veterans Recently Separated from the Military

T0308520

For more information on this publication, visit **www.rand.org/t/RRA3304-1**.

About RAND

RAND is a research organization that develops solutions to public policy challenges to help make communities throughout the world safer and more secure, healthier and more prosperous. RAND is nonprofit, nonpartisan, and committed to the public interest. To learn more about RAND, visit www.rand.org.

Research Integrity

Our mission to help improve policy and decisionmaking through research and analysis is enabled through our core values of quality and objectivity and our unwavering commitment to the highest level of integrity and ethical behavior. To help ensure our research and analysis are rigorous, objective, and nonpartisan, we subject our research publications to a robust and exacting quality-assurance process; avoid both the appearance and reality of financial and other conflicts of interest through staff training, project screening, and a policy of mandatory disclosure; and pursue transparency in our research engagements through our commitment to the open publication of our research findings and recommendations, disclosure of the source of funding of published research, and policies to ensure intellectual independence. For more information, visit www.rand.org/about/research-integrity.

RAND's publications do not necessarily reflect the opinions of its research clients and sponsors.

Published by the RAND Corporation, Santa Monica, Calif.
© 2024 RAND Corporation
RAND® is a registered trademark.

Library of Congress Cataloging-in-Publication Data is available for this publication.
ISBN: 978-1-9774-1408-3

Limited Print and Electronic Distribution Rights

About This Report

This report presents the findings of a survey of recently discharged or separated service members residing in New York state. The study aimed to assess veterans' needs by understanding the health and well-being of recently discharged or separated veterans, identifying barriers to accessing services, and learning about their experiences with health care provided through the Department of Veterans Affairs (VA). The results offer critical information that can inform policy and practice changes to improve awareness of, access to, and use of needed services among veterans living in New York.

This work was funded by the New York Health Foundation.

The findings of this report will be of particular interest to policymakers, veterans' advocacy groups, and health care providers who are involved in the design and delivery of services for veterans. Additionally, researchers and academics focusing on social and economic well-being, public health, and veteran affairs will find the data and conclusions useful for further studies.

Social and Behavioral Policy Program

RAND Social and Economic Well-Being is a division of RAND that seeks to actively improve the health and social and economic well-being of populations and communities throughout the world. This research was conducted in the Social and Behavioral Policy Program within RAND Social and Economic Well-Being. The program focuses on such topics as risk factors and prevention programs, social safety net programs and other social supports, poverty, aging, disability, child and youth health and well-being, and quality of life, as well as other policy concerns that are influenced by social and behavioral actions and systems that affect well-being. For more information, email sbp@rand.org.

RAND Epstein Family Veterans Policy Research Institute

The RAND Epstein Family Veterans Policy Research Institute is dedicated to conducting innovative, evidence-based research and analysis to improve the lives of those who have served in the U.S. military. Building on decades of interdisciplinary expertise at the RAND Corporation, the institute prioritizes creative, equitable, and inclusive solutions and interventions that meet the needs of diverse veteran populations while engaging and empowering those who support them. For more information about the RAND Epstein Family Veterans Policy Research Institute, visit veterans.rand.org. Questions about this report or about the RAND Epstein Family Veterans Policy Research Institute should be directed to veteranspolicy@rand.org.

Acknowledgments

This project would not have been possible without the support and assistance of many people. We are grateful to our project officer, Derek Coy, and other staff at the New York Health Foundation who provided important input on survey content and sampling procedures. We are extremely grateful to the respondents for investing their time in completing the survey and sharing their experiences and insights. Finally, we would like to thank our quality assurance reviewers, Sara Kintzle and Megan Schuler; their thoughtful and constructive comments significantly improved the report. Any remaining errors are the sole responsibility of the authors.

Summary

Over the past decade, there has been increased awareness that U.S. military veterans often grapple with significant mental and physical health issues related to their service. In response, many policies and programs have been put in place to support veterans and improve access to needed services. Despite these efforts, prevalence rates for physical and mental health problems and concerns about the health and overall well-being of veterans remain high. Because the specific needs of veterans and the barriers to accessing care likely differ across areas, data at the state level are critical for tailoring policies and programs to make them more effective.

This study focuses on veterans in New York, specifically individuals discharged or separated from the military between January 2018 and January 2023. RAND researchers fielded and analyzed responses from a survey of 1,122 veterans (see the box) designed to assess the mental and physical health of this cohort of veterans and their access to, and experiences with, health care and other veteran benefits.

> **Recently Separated Veterans in New York: A Closer Look at the Study Sample**
>
> Of the 1,122 recently separated veterans living in New York who participated in the study approximately
>
> - 39 percent were under age 35
> - 62 percent were under age 45
> - 15 percent were women and nearly 40 percent were non-White
> - half had a college degree or higher
> - 70 percent were employed either full- or part-time
> - 51 percent served in the Army, although individuals from all services participated in the study.

Findings

Many surveyed New York veterans face mental health challenges. Figure S.1 summarizes the primary challenges faced by New York veterans. Those with combat deployments had lower rates of depression but higher rates of posttraumatic stress disorder (PTSD) compared with those without combat deployments. Veterans in the survey reported suicidal thoughts twice as much than the estimates for the general New York adult population.

FIGURE S.1

Measures of Mental Health Status Among Recently Separated Veterans in New York

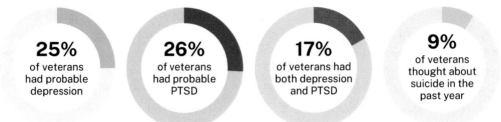

25% of veterans had probable depression

26% of veterans had probable PTSD

17% of veterans had both depression and PTSD

9% of veterans thought about suicide in the past year

Many also face physical health challenges. Approximately 20 percent rated their health as "fair" or "poor." This proportion is higher than estimates for the general population ages 18 to 54, but like those for ages 55 to 64. In addition, nearly two-thirds reported having a Department of Veterans Affairs (VA) disability rating. This suggests veterans experience a greater health burden than the general population of the same age.

Many face challenges getting enough food. Approximately one-quarter of respondents experienced food insecurity in the past year.

Most have some form of health insurance, but this does not necessarily translate into health care access. Ninety-seven percent of respondents had some form of health insurance coverage and over three-quarters can access care through VA, but only 70 percent reported having a "usual" source of care—that is, a primary professional or location that they usually go to when they need health care services.

Many have unmet physical and mental health care needs. Figure S.2 breaks this finding down into percentages and the top three barriers to care in each category. The rate of unmet need for mental health services is even higher (39 percent) among those with a probable mental health diagnosis.

Most view VA health care services positively. Respondents reported that they had good experiences in both VA facilities and those in the community paid for by VA. Veterans noted that it was easier to schedule convenient appointments with community facilities but that health providers in VA facilities were more likely to understand military culture and the unique health challenges faced by veterans.

A significant proportion reported a preference for community providers over military or VA facilities. The most common reasons included easier access (48.5 percent), better perceived quality of care (43.9 percent), and established relationships with existing providers (39.5 percent).

FIGURE S.2
Unmet Needs for and Barriers to Care

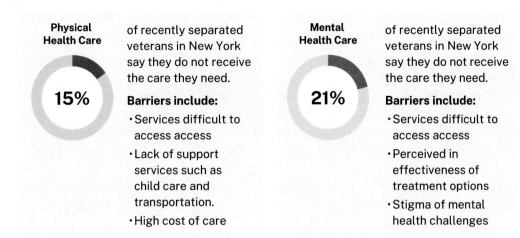

Physical Health Care

15%

of recently separated veterans in New York say they do not receive the care they need.

Barriers include:
- Services difficult to access access
- Lack of support services such as child care and transportation.
- High cost of care

Mental Health Care

21%

of recently separated veterans in New York say they do not receive the care they need.

Barriers include:
- Services difficult to access access
- Perceived in effectiveness of treatment options
- Stigma of mental health challenges

Many see veterans' benefits helpful but don't use them. Almost 46 percent of survey respondents said that veteran housing assistance and loans are helpful, yet only 20 percent used them. Similarly, job training was seen as helpful (34 percent), while fewer had accessed it (10 percent).

Comparison with 2010 Needs Assessment of Veterans Living in New York

The current study builds on a similar needs assessment conducted in 2010 among recently separated veterans in New York. The comparison of the current survey results with our 2010 study reveals several notable differences in the health and well-being of veterans living in New York. The current cohort of veterans reports higher rates of mental health problems, with 24.5 percent screening positive for depression and 25.5 percent for PTSD, compared with 16 percent for each condition in the prior study. This could represent a higher prevalence of mental health problems, greater awareness of and reduced stigma around mental health, and/or differences in the demographics of the samples. Additionally, the current sample shows more disability, with 62.8 percent having a VA or military disability rating versus 31 percent in 2010, and a higher average percentage disability rating (68.5 percent vs. 38 percent). Despite these increases, the proportion reporting unmet mental health needs remained consistent at around 21 percent. However, the barriers to accessing mental health services have shifted, with more veterans in the current sample reporting not knowing how to find the proper services and believing that the care would not be effective.

Recommendations

Enhance access to and use of mental health services. Consider making available more health professionals trained to work with veterans, integrating mental health services into community and primary care settings, and addressing mental health stigma through innovative media campaigns to improve care uptake.

Continue to prioritize veteran-specific suicide prevention programs. Continued commitment to policies, programs, and research efforts in this area is critical. These include improving the quality and accessibility of data on veteran suicide risk and mortality and on expanding and evaluating veteran-specific approaches to suicide prevention and crisis intervention.

Support veterans' ability to access both VA-based and community-based health care services. Maintaining choice and access to the different care settings is needed to meet the diverse needs of veterans across New York.

Address logistical barriers veterans face to accessing needed health care. Transportation to appointments, more flexible appointment times and locations, and providing additional support through free resources such as the NYS [New York State] Veterans mobile app could help.

Improve and expand outreach and awareness about benefits and services. This could involve partnerships with community organizations and targeted information campaigns advertising existing VA outreach events and services to reach a broader audience, and should include information about all challenges facing veterans, including food insecurity.

Consider the growing diversity of the veteran population. Service providers should receive ongoing training on equity and cultural competence to meet the needs of the current and future veteran population. Programs that explicitly address the unique challenges faced by veteran women, LGBTQ+ veterans, and those from racial and ethnic minority backgrounds are and will be necessary going forward.

Contents

Figures and Tables

Figures

Tables

CHAPTER 1

Introduction

Over the past decade, the experiences and composition of U.S. military veterans have notably changed. Today's veterans are younger and more diverse in terms of gender, race, and ethnicity (Robinson et al., 2023). The proportion of veteran women has increased from 7 percent of pre-9/11 veterans to 17 percent of post-9/11 veterans. The proportion of non-Hispanic Black veterans has increased from 11 percent of pre-9/11 veterans to 15 percent of post-9/11 veterans, and the proportion of Hispanic/Latino veterans has increased from 5.7 percent of pre-9/11 veterans to 13 percent of post-9/11 veterans (Robinson et al., 2023). The conclusion of Operation Enduring Freedom (OEF) and Operation Iraqi Freedom (OIF)—conflicts that deployed over 1.9 million service members and were characterized by repeated and extended deployments (Institute of Medicine, 2010)—has heightened awareness of the invisible injuries of war, including posttraumatic stress disorder (PTSD), depression, substance misuse, and traumatic brain injury (Tanielian et al., 2008). The coronavirus disease 2019 (COVID-19) pandemic further affected the daily lives and interactions of both veterans and nonveterans, adding an additional layer of stress and uncertainty to an already complex landscape.

Over the last ten years, there have been important policy changes that expanded eligibility and access to the care veterans receive. Numerous policy commitments and strategies have been implemented to increase access to health care within Veterans Health Administration (VHA) services and in the community. The Veterans' Access to Care Through Choice, Accountability, and Transparency Act, also known as the Veterans Choice Act, was passed in 2014 (Pub. L. 113-146, 2014), establishing the Veterans Choice Program and widening the eligibility criteria for veterans to access "community care" (i.e., care paid for by VHA benefits but delivered by medical providers outside of the VHA). The subsequent John S. McCain III, Daniel K. Akaka, and Samuel R. Johnson VA Maintaining Internal Systems and Strengthening Integrated Outside Networks Act, also known as the VA MISSION Act, passed in 2018 (Pub. L. 115-182, 2018), further expanded the Department of Veterans Affairs (VA) and VHA services by broadening eligibility criteria for community care and established a more consolidated network of community care options. In 2019, the Commander John Scott Hannon Veterans Mental Health Care Improvement Act (Pub. L. 116-177, 2020) was passed to broaden veteran access to mental health care and suicide prevention services through strategies such as increasing access to telehealth treatment among veterans in rural areas, integrating behavioral health services into VA health care, and increasing funding for veteran mental health research, mental health clinician training, and innovative pilot programs. The

2022 Sergeant First Class Heath Robinson Honoring Our Promise to Address Comprehensive Toxics (PACT) Act (Pub. L. 117-168, 2022) increased the number of medical conditions presumed to be service-connected, thereby further expanding available coverage for health care and disability benefits (Chari, Salazar, and Skrabala, 2024).

Despite these efforts to enhance access to care for veterans, prevalence rates for physical and mental health problems and concerns about the health and overall well-being of veterans remain high. Compared with nonveteran U.S. adults, veterans face higher rates of mental health disorders and suicide mortality. Suicide ranks as the second-leading cause of death among veterans under 45 years of age in the United States and rates of suicides among veterans are rising faster than nonveterans (VA, 2023). Estimates of the prevalence of depression and PTSD among veterans vary greatly across studies. A recent meta-analysis found a 20-percent prevalence rate of depression among veterans across data from 40 studies (Moradi, Dowran, and Sepandi, 2021). VA data suggests that as many as 15 percent of OIF and OEF veterans experience PTSD symptoms in a given year (Na, Schnurr, and Pietrzak, 2023). Additionally, during the height of the COVID-19 pandemic from 2020 to 2021, veterans experienced more mental health concerns than nonveterans, including more frequent alcohol use, stress, loneliness, and suicidal ideation (Li et al., 2023).

This report is the second research study completed by RAND for the New York Health Foundation aimed at better understanding the needs of recently separated veterans living in the state of New York. RAND published the first report in 2011, which was based on integrated findings from qualitative interviews and quantitative surveys with OEF and OIF veterans and their families living in New York conducted in 2010 (Farmer et al., 2011). Results from the 2010 sample suggested that 22 percent of veterans in New York met criteria for a probable mental health diagnosis as defined in the *Diagnostic and Statistical Manual of Mental Disorders, Fourth Edition (DSM-IV)*, based on their report of symptoms in the past 30 days. Additionally, 16 percent of the sample screened positive for PTSD, compared with the general population prevalence estimate of 2 percent, and 16 percent screened positive for depression, compared with the general population prevalence estimates at the time of 4 to 7 percent. Further, veterans in the 2010 sample reported worse physical health outcomes and higher rates of unemployment compared with the overall New York adult population (Farmer et al., 2011).

National-level research studies on veteran characteristics (e.g., demographics, socioeconomic status, health status) and service utilization shed light on the current state of veterans generally but may not accurately capture the unique needs of veterans living in a particular state. Additionally, many studies rely solely on VHA data and do not represent the health care needs of veterans who are not eligible for VHA services or who are opting to seek services elsewhere. Therefore, collecting data from representative, community-dwelling samples of veterans, including those who do not receive VHA care, is of the utmost importance to understand the needs of veterans living in New York and to inform state-level policies and resource allocation.

The study reported here was designed to assess the needs of a cohort of veterans who recently separated from the military and live in New York. Specifically, this study evaluated (1) the mental and physical health of this cohort of veterans; and (2) their access to, and experiences with, health care. To a lesser degree, we also explored additional factors affecting veteran health, well-being, and service use, such as employment, income, and food insecurity. We collected survey data from a random sample of veterans residing in New York who were recently separated from the military. Our sample included both those who use VHA services and those who do not. The report is organized into three chapters and an appendix. Chapter 1 provides a brief introduction; Chapter 2 summarizes our survey design and data collection methodology and presents results; and the final chapter discusses the implications of our research and policy and practice recommendations. Additional details about survey methods can be found in the appendix.

Survey Methods and Results

Survey Methods

The objective of this research was to collect data from a random sample of recently separated veterans residing in New York. This section provides a high-level overview of our procedures; additional detail is provided in the Appendix. The data that served as the basis for our sample were obtained through a request for names and addresses (RONA) from VA. RAND requested information for all veterans that separated from the military in the previous five years (between January 2018 and January 2023) and reported a New York address at the time of separation. The sample included all veterans who met the parameters regardless of discharge status or whether they have used any VA services since discharge, resulting in a total of 30,194 records.

We drew a random sample of 20,561 names from the universe of records. Two databases—V12 and LexisNexis—were used to update addresses and append emails when available. Individuals no longer residing in New York state were then excluded, leaving a total of 12,516 individuals in the sample. We received 1,171 fully or partially completed surveys from people meeting eligibility criteria (i.e., currently live in New York, have served in the military, and are not currently on active duty), achieving a response rate of 12.7 percent.[1] We excluded 49 partially completed surveys that did not contain sufficient data for analysis. The final analysis sample included 1,122 veterans.[2] All respondents who completed the survey were offered a $25 gift card as a token of appreciation for their time and input.

Data collection was conducted in two stages: a pilot test and the main survey. The pilot test aimed to identify the most effective survey fielding approach by testing five different methods, each involving approximately 250 individuals. These methods varied in terms of the content of the mailings (e.g., push-to-web letters, hard copies of the survey) and the means of delivery (e.g., United States Postal Service [USPS], FedEx). The push-to-web letters included a

---

[1] This was calculated using the American Association of Public Opinion Research (AAPOR) Response Rate 4 Calculator. For specific details, see AAPOR, undated.

[2] The sample does include some people who have separated from the military but who are currently in the National Guard or the reserves. The Appendix provides additional detail on these individuals, how they differ from others in the sample, and the rationale for their inclusion.

URL and QR code along with a unique PIN for respondents to access the web-based survey. Each arm of the pilot test received two mailings, and for some arms, a hardcopy of the survey was included in the second mailing in place of a push-to-web letter. The pilot test took place in November and December 2023, and the results helped refine the methodology for the main survey.

For the main survey, respondents received USPS push-to-web letters for the first and second mailings, as this method was found to be the least expensive and achieved a comparable response rate with other methods. In addition, up to five email reminders were sent to respondents with email addresses on file to encourage their participation. Data collection for the main survey occurred in February and March 2024.

We developed nonresponse weights using urbanicity and proxies for demographic characteristics, including race/ethnicity, gender, and age—these proxies are determined for respondents and nonrespondents using name and address only. The weights were used to conduct descriptive analyses of the survey data that reflect the full population of recently discharged veterans in New York, not just those who responded to the survey.

The survey gathered extensive information on various aspects of recently separated veterans' lives, including their physical and mental health needs, service use, and sociodemographic characteristics. The survey measures were designed to align with those used in the 2010 study of veterans in New York (Farmer et al., 2011). All survey materials and procedures were reviewed and approved by the RAND Human Subjects Protection Committee, and respondents provided written informed consent, ensuring ethical standards were maintained throughout the study.

Survey Results

In this section, we report results of descriptive analyses of the survey data. For all measures, we report results across the full, applicable sample. For some measures, however, we also report results for particular subgroups of interest. To provide context for the key results related to health, well-being, and health care access, we also report, where available, estimates from the literature for the general population of adults and for other veteran samples. We also provide comparisons with the 2010 study of veterans in New York (Farmer et al., 2011). These comparisons provide useful context for the results but are based on populations that may differ in important ways from the sample of recently separated veterans in New York (e.g., samples with different age and gender distributions). So, while they provide important and useful information, it is difficult to say whether differences in the estimates between the current sample and those reported in the literature reflect differences in the underlying prevalence and/or the composition of the populations being studied.

Sociodemographic Characteristics and Military Experience

Sociodemographic Characteristics

Table 2.1 presents the demographic and socioeconomic characteristics of veterans in the sample. We report means (or proportions) and the 95-percent confidence intervals (CIs). Due to the nature of the underlying population—veterans recently separated from the military—respondents were relatively young compared with the full population of veterans, with over one-third between the ages of 25 and 34 and the vast majority (91.6 percent) younger than 65. In contrast, only about one-half of the full population of veterans in the United States is younger than 65 (Vespa, 2023). This difference in age composition makes comparisons between the current sample and the full population of veterans difficult to interpret as differences in outcomes can reflect both differences in age and actual differences in the prevalence of the outcome.

Approximately 15 percent of recently separated veterans were women and nearly 40 percent reported a race/ethnicity other than White (13.0 percent Black, 16.5 percent Hispanic, and 8.5 percent "Other"). About half of recently separated veterans have a college degree or higher and 70.5 percent were employed (63 percent full-time and 7.5 percent part-time). Approximately 20 percent of recently separated veterans live in New York City, 62.8 percent live in an urban area other than New York City, and 15.7 percent live in a rural area (i.e., outside of a metropolitan statistical area [MSA]). While 36.7 percent reported household income of $100,000 or above, there was a nontrivial proportion that reported income of less than $40,000 (4.3 percent with income less than $20,000 and 10.9 percent with income between $20,000 and $40,000). Using information on income and household size, we estimate that between approximately 3.5 and 6.4 percent of veterans in our sample had incomes below the poverty line (Office of the Assistant Secretary for Planning and Evaluation, 2024).[3] This is lower than the 11.7-percent poverty rate estimated for the general population of adults (aged 18–64) in 2022 (Benson, 2023), likely due to the high rate of employment in the sample.

Compared with the sample from the prior study (Farmer et al., 2011), the current sample is older (38.6 percent vs. 54 percent under age 35), more diverse in terms or race and gender (62 percent vs. 73 percent White; 14.7 percent vs. 11 percent female), and more educated (49.7 vs. 33 percent with a college degree or higher), but similar on other dimensions such as employment (70.5 percent vs. 72 percent currently employed either full- or part-time).

---

[3] The income bands reported in the survey do not match up precisely with the poverty line income thresholds. We therefore calculate the estimate two ways. For a lower-bound estimate, we only considered a household in poverty if the whole income band was below the threshold for a household of their size. For example, consider a respondent with a household of three people and reported income in the range $20,000 to less than $30,000. The poverty threshold for a three-person household is $25,800. Because we do not know whether this respondent's income is above or below the threshold, we did not designate them as in poverty. For an upper-bound estimate, we considered a household in poverty if the poverty threshold for a household of their size was within the reported income band.

TABLE 2.1

Sociodemographic Characteristics of Recently Separated Veterans in New York

Characteristic	Percentage	95% CI LL	95% CI UL
Age			
18–24	3.5	2.2	4.7
25–34	35.1	31.9	38.2
35–44	23.8	21.1	26.6
45–54	16.1	13.7	18.5
55–64	13.1	11.2	15.0
65+	8.4	6.9	10.0
Gender			
Female	14.7	12.4	17.1
Race/Ethnicity			
Black	13.0	10.4	15.6
Hispanic	16.5	13.8	19.2
White	62.0	58.7	65.3
Other	8.5	6.8	10.2
Education Level			
High school diploma	29.1	26.1	32.1
Associates degree	21.2	18.5	23.8
College degree or higher	49.8	46.5	53.0
Relationship Status			
Married	59.0	55.9	62.2
Employment Status			
Employed full-time (35+ hours per week)	63.0	59.8	66.2
Employed part-time (<35 hours per week)	7.5	5.8	9.2
Unemployed	7.8	5.7	9.8
Not in the labor force	18.6	16.2	21.1
Other	3.1	1.8	4.5

TABLE 2.1—Continued

Characteristic	Percentage	95% CI LL	95% CI UL
Income			
Less than $20,000	4.4	3.0	5.7
$20,000 to less than $40,000	10.9	8.7	13.1
$40,000 to less than $50,000	10.5	8.2	12.7
$50,000 to less than $75,000	17.6	14.9	20.3
$75,000 to less than $100,000	20.0	17.3	22.7
$100,000 or more	36.7	33.6	39.8
Geography			
Reside in rural area	15.7	12.8	18.7
Reside in New York City	21.5	18.8	24.1
Current Military Status			
Separated from the military	47.3	44.1	50.6
Retired from the military	41.9	38.6	45.1
Serving in the National Guard or reserves	10.8	8.8	12.7

NOTE: LL = lower limit; UL = upper limit.

Military Experience

Among respondents, 47.3 percent reported being separated from the military, 41.9 percent reported they had retired from the military, and 10.8 percent reported they were currently serving in the National Guard or reserves. Among the veterans that reported being separated from the military, 97.2 percent reported their discharge status as honorable.[4] Figure 2.1 shows the distribution of respondents across the branches of service. The proportions ranged from a high of 50.9 percent (95-percent CI: 47.7–54.1) having served most recently in the Army to 1.2 percent (95-percent CI: 0.6–1.8) in the Coast Guard. Only one respondent reported the Space Force as the last branch that they served in (not shown).[5]

Table 2.2 shows the distribution across the highest military pay grade achieved by respondents. Pay grades for enlisted personnel and officers are given by E1–E9, and O1–O10, respectively, with higher numbers meaning higher pay. The ranks associated with these pay grades differ across branches of service. Nearly 80 percent of respondents separated from the military as enlisted personnel (E1–E9), 27.6 percent with E1–E4, and 51.5 percent with E5–E9 as their

---

[4] "Honorable" includes two response options: honorable discharge and general discharge under honorable conditions.

[5] The study sample does not include veterans of the U.S. Public Health Service Corps or the National Oceanic and Atmospheric Administration Commissioned Officer Corps.

FIGURE 2.1

Branch of Service

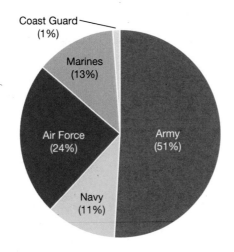

TABLE 2.2

Highest Military Pay Grade Achieved

Military Pay Grade	Percentage	95% CI LL	95% CI UL
E1–E4	27.7	24.6	30.7
E5–E9	51.5	48.3	54.7
O1–O3	6.9	5.3	8.5
O4 or above	13.5	11.5	15.5
I don't remember	0.5	0.1	0.8

NOTE: LL = lower limit; UL = upper limit.

highest pay grade achieved. Length of service is high in the current sample relative to the general veteran population. The mean number of years served in the military was 14.7 (95-percent CI: 14.0–15.4) compared with approximately four years in the full population of veterans.[6]

Just over 60 percent of respondents (60.1 percent; 95-percent CI: 57.0–63.4) reported that they deployed on a combat mission during their military service. Among those who deployed, the average number of deployments was 2.2 (95-percent CI: 2.1–2.3) and the median was 2.

Compared with the prior study, the distribution across branches of service and the rank at time of discharge are similar (Farmer et al., 2011). One key difference is that the prior study focused on individuals who had deployed, whereas the current sample includes people who never deployed to a combat operation during their military service.

---

[6] Estimate of average years of service is from the authors' analysis of the 2023 Current Population Survey, Veteran Supplement; see IPUMS Current Population Survey (CPS), undated.

Health and Well-Being

Mental Health

Using a four-week look-back period of symptoms, 24.6 percent and 25.5 percent of respondents screened positive for depression and PTSD, respectively (see Table 2.3). The co-occurrence of depression and PTSD was common among respondents in our sample, with 16.5 percent of respondents screening positive for both.

The proportion with probable depression in our sample was somewhat higher than a recent estimate of 18.5 percent for the general adult population (Villarroel and Terlizzi, 2020) and a 20-percent prevalence estimate among veterans from a recent meta-analysis of over 40 studies (Moradi, Dowran, and Sepandi, 2021). The proportion with probable PTSD in our sample was substantially higher than estimates for the general adult population, where about 5 percent are estimated to have PTSD in any given year (Goldstein et al., 2016). The rates estimated in this sample were also higher than estimates from other published VA data indicating that approximately 15 percent of veterans of OIF or OEF experience symptoms of PTSD in a given year (Na, Schnurr, and Pietrzak, 2023). The rates of probable mental health diagnoses are higher in the current sample than what was found in the 2010 study, where 16 percent of the sample screened positive for PTSD and 16 percent screened positive for depression (Farmer et al., 2011).

We looked at probable mental health diagnoses by deployment status because military service during the eras of OEF and OIF often involved repeated and extended deployments (Institute of Medicine, 2010) and there has been increased awareness of the invisible injuries of combat, including PTSD and depression (Tanielian et al., 2008). We grouped respondents

TABLE 2.3

Rates of Probable Depression, Probable PTSD, and Suicidal Ideation

Condition	Percentage	95% CI LL	95% CI UL
Probable depression, past four weeks	24.6	21.7	27.5
Probable PTSD, past four weeks	25.6	22.5	28.6
Comorbidity			
No depression or PTSD	67.0	63.8	70.26
Only depression	7.5	5.8	9.3
Only PTSD	9.0	6.8	11.1
Both depression and PTSD	16.5	13.9	19.1
Suicidal ideation in past year	8.7	6.7	10.8
Made plans to die by suicide	11.7	5.0	18.4
Attempted suicide	0.8	0.0	2.4

NOTE: Probable depression and probable PTSD are measured over a four-week look-back period; suicidal ideation is measured over the past year. LL = lower limit; UL = upper limit.

into three categories: those who never deployed to a combat operation, those that deployed one to three times, and those that deployed four or more times. Respondents that had experienced four or more combat deployments had significantly lower rates of probable depression (10.6 percent, 95-percent CI: 4.4–16.8) than respondents who deployed one to three times (23.7 percent; 95-percent CI: 19.9–27.4) and respondents who never deployed (28.6 percent, 95-percent CI: 23.4–33.9). For PTSD, respondents who deployed one to three times had the highest rates of probable PTSD (30.2 percent, 95-percent CI: 25.8–34.6) compared with those who never deployed (20.8 percent, 95-percent CI: 15.9–25.8) and those who deployed four or more times (19.0 percent, 95-percent CI: 10.7–27.2) (see Figure 2.2).

Suicide

Among respondents, 8.7 percent reported having had suicidal thoughts in the last year (see Table 2.3). This is more than two times the prevalence of 3.7 percent found among the general adult population in New York state in 2019 (Ivey-Stephenson et al., 2022). However, it is lower than a recent estimate of 15 percent of veterans having had suicidal thoughts from a large meta-analysis (Moradi, Dowran, and Sepandi, 2021). Among respondents who experienced suicidal thoughts, 11.7 percent had made plans to die by suicide and 0.8 percent reported having made a suicide attempt.

FIGURE 2.2

Mental Health Status in Past Four Weeks by Combat Deployment Status

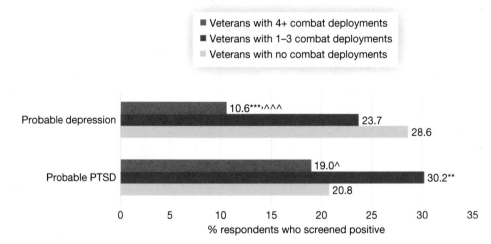

NOTE: *$p<0.05$, **$p<0.01$, ***$p<0.001$ from a chi-squared test of differences in the estimated proportion of respondents that screened positive for a probable mental health condition, compared with no combat.
^ $p<0.05$, ^^ $p<0.01$, ^^^ $p<0.001$ from a chi-squared test of differences in the estimated proportion of respondents that screened positive for a probable mental health condition, compared with 1–3 combat deployments.

Substance Use

Almost one-third of respondents reported no alcohol consumption in the past 30 days (see Table 2.4). A similar proportion, however, reported at least one binge-drinking episode in the past 30 days, and just over 10 percent reported frequent binge drinking (i.e., five or more binge-drinking episodes) in the past 30 days. The proportion of respondents reporting at least one binge-drinking episode is close to estimates for a similarly aged adult population: the rate is 30.5 percent and 29.2 percent of adults between the ages of 19 and 30 and 35 and 50, respectively (Patrick et al., 2023). The rate of past-month binge drinking among the current sample (28.7 percent) is somewhat higher than the 22.9 percent reported by a nationally representative survey of the U.S. veteran population over the period 2015–2019 (Robinson et al., 2023), but this is likely due in part to differences in the age distribution of the two samples. Compared with the 2010 study, the current sample reports lower rates of alcohol use overall (71 percent vs. 78 percent reporting some alcohol use in 2010) and of binge drinking (10.6 percent vs. 16 percent reporting frequent binge drinking in 2010) (Farmer et al., 2011).

The use of marijuana and other cannabis products is legal in New York for adults over the age of 21 (see NYC Health, undated). Among respondents, 20.7 percent reported use of a cannabis product in the past year (see Table 2.5). This rate is lower than recent estimates from similarly aged adult populations, where 43.6 percent of adults ages 19 to 30 and 27.9 percent of adults ages 35 to 50 reported past year cannabis use (Patrick et al., 2023). However, as might be expected, this rate is higher than recent national estimates showing 10.2 percent of veterans using cannabis in the past year since not all states have legalized marijuana use (Robinson et al., 2023).

The rates of illegal drug use and misuse of prescription drugs among respondents were much lower than the rates for cannabis: 1.3 percent and 3.3 percent, respectively. The rate of

TABLE 2.4

Rates of Alcohol Abstinence and Binge Drinking in the Past 30 Days

Alcohol Use	Percentage	95% CI LL	95% CI UL
Abstinence from alcohol consumption	29.0	26.2	31.8
At least one binge-drinking episode	28.7	25.7	31.6
Frequent binge drinking (5+ times)	10.5	8.6	12.4

NOTE: LL = lower limit; UL = upper limit.

TABLE 2.5

Rates of Substance Use in the Past Year

Substance	Percentage	95% CI LL	95% CI UL
Marijuana or cannabis products	20.7	18.0	23.4
Illegal drugs (e.g., cocaine, heroin, amphetamines)	1.3	0.6	2.0
Prescription medication misuse	3.3	2.0	4.6

NOTE: LL = lower limit; UL = upper limit.

illicit drug use, 1.3 percent, is substantially lower in this sample of veterans than in the general adult population where 17.4 percent of adults ages 19 to 30 and 11.9 percent of adults ages 35 to 50 reported using illegal drugs in the past year (Patrick et al., 2023). Further, the rate of illicit drug use among respondents was lower than the 5.5-percent rate of illicit drug use seen in a nationally representative sample of veterans (Robinson et al., 2023). The rates of illegal drug use were similar to what was found in the 2010 study (1.3 percent vs. 2 percent in 2010). The key difference is that because of legalization many more in the current study report the use of marijuana or cannabis products (20.7 percent vs. 7 percent in 2010) (Farmer et al., 2011).

Physical Health

Table 2.6 presents information about the physical health of recently separated veterans. Approximately 40 percent of respondents reported their health status as "very good" or "excellent" and 20 percent reported "fair" or "poor." This proportion is higher than estimates for the general population of adults ages 18 to 44 (8.4 percent) and 45 to 54 (15.3 percent) reporting "fair" or "poor" health and similar to the rate for the population ages 55 to 64 (21.7 percent) (National Center for Health Statistics, 2023). It is somewhat lower than estimates for veterans enrolled in VA health care, where 26 percent report their health as "fair" or "poor" (VA, 2022). On the Physical Functioning and Role Limitations Due to Physical Health subscales of the 36-Item Short Form Health Survey (SF-36; Ware et al., 1993), respondents reported lower scores than norms adjusted for the age and gender distribution of our sample (scores range between 0 and 100 with higher scores meaning better physical functioning). The

TABLE 2.6

Physical Health Characteristics of Recently Separated Veterans in New York

Health Characteristics	Percentage or Mean	95% CI LL	95% CI UL
General health status			
Excellent	9.4	7.7	11.2
Very good	30.2	27.3	33.1
Good	39.5	36.3	42.6
Fair	16.7	14.3	19.2
Poor	4.2	2.6	5.9
Physical functioning score (mean)	77.3	75.5	79.1
Role limitations score (mean)	71.2	69.0	73.5
Possible health condition related to exposure to toxic chemicals	43.5	39.4	47.5
Ever rated as disabled or partially disabled by military or VA	62.8	59.6	65.9
Average disability rating among the disabled (mean)	68.5	66.0	71.0

NOTE: The age and gender adjusted norm for the general population is 87.5 for the physical functioning score and 84.8 for the role limitations score. LL = lower limit; UL = upper limit.

average physical functioning score among respondents was 77.3 compared with an adjusted norm of 87.5. The average role limitations score among respondents was 71.2 compared with an adjusted norm of 84.8. These scores are approximately 0.2 (for role limitations) to 0.3 (for physical functioning) standard deviations below the age- and sex-adjusted norms, which is considered a small to medium difference (J. Cohen, 2013). This finding aligns with other studies that have shown veterans have worse health outcomes than nonveterans (Betancourt et al., 2023). It is also similar to findings from the 2010 study (Farmer et al., 2011).

The lower scores on the physical functioning and role limitations scales may reflect the high rate of disability in the sample. Over 60 percent reported being rated as fully or partially disabled by the military or VA. Among those with disability ratings, the average disability rating was 68.5 percent. The level of disability in the current sample is substantially higher than was found in the 2010 study, where 31 percent reported being rated as disabled and the average disability rating among those was 38 percent (Farmer et al., 2011).

In addition, nearly half of respondents reported they believe they have a health condition related to exposure to toxic chemicals during their military service. This significant proportion may be indicative of the growing public awareness of the health risks associated with common service-related exposures to toxic chemicals (e.g., burn pits) that led to the passing of the PACT Act in 2022 (Chari, Salazar, and Skrabala, 2024). As of July 2024, VA had screened over 5.6 million veterans for potential toxic exposures, with over 2.5 million (44.8 percent) reporting at least one potential exposure, pointing to the importance of timely detection and treatment of health conditions that can result from such exposures (VA, 2024).

Firearm Safety

Over 40 percent of respondents reported keeping firearms in or around their home (see Table 2.7). Among those, 27.1 percent reported their guns are loaded, and 36.4 percent reported that the guns are unlocked. These estimates are generally in line with recent estimates for the adult population in several states (Friar et al., 2024), where the proportion with guns in or around the household ranged from 18 to 50 percent, depending on the state (Alaska had the highest rate and California had the lowest).[7] The proportion where the guns were loaded ranged

TABLE 2.7
Firearm Use and Safety

	All Veterans		
	Percentage	95% CI LL	95% CI UL
Any firearms kept in or around home	42.3	39.1	45.5
Firearms in or around home are loaded	27.0	22.5	31.4
Firearms in or around home are unlocked	36.7	26.7	46.6

NOTE: LL = lower limit; UL = upper limit.

_____

[7] States included in the study are Alaska, California, Minnesota, Nevada, New Mexico, North Carolina, Ohio, and Oklahoma.

among states from 20 to 40 percent and unlocked ranged among states from 49 to 57 percent (Friar et al., 2024). Rates of firearm ownership and unsafe storage practices among respondents were similar, although slightly lower, than those reported by U.S. veteran adults in the 2015 National Firearms Survey, where 45 percent of veterans owned a firearm and 33 percent stored at least one firearm in the home loaded and unlocked (Simonetti et al., 2018).

Food Insecurity

Social factors, such as adequate access to nutritious food, play an important role in determining health. Using the Hunger Vital Sign (Hager et al., 2010), approximately one-quarter of respondents indicated that they had experienced food insecurity during the past year (25.7 percent; 95-percent CI: 22.7–29.0). This rate is approximately twice the national average of 12.8 percent in 2022; however, the national estimate is based on a more detailed measure of food insecurity so may not be directly comparable (Rabbitt et al., 2023). A recent study looking specifically at food insecurity among working-age veterans found rates similar to the national average at 11.1 percent (Rabbitt and Smith, 2021). Other estimates for veteran populations range from 6 to 24 percent (Dubowitz, 2021). The higher rate found in this study may be attributable in part to differences in how food insecurity is measured across studies and differences in the cost of living in New York relative to other areas. Regardless of what drives the difference, a substantial portion of veterans in New York were concerned about having enough money for food at some point during the past year.

Findings are consistent with previous research showing that, among veterans, those who are younger and who have recently left active-duty military service (akin to the current sample) are at higher risk of food insecurity (Brostow, Gunzburger, and Thomas, 2017; London and Heflin, 2015; Widome et al., 2015). Reports of food insecurity in the current sample may speak to a lack of access to needed food assistance programs. Recent research on food-insecure veteran populations showcased the underenrollment of income-eligible veterans in federal food assistance programs such as the Supplemental Nutrition Assistance Program (SNAP). Recent research identified barriers to participation including lack of knowledge about SNAP and stigma related to use of such services. The research highlighted how veteran participation in VA disability benefits programs may also render some veterans ineligible for SNAP assistance based on their income, despite ongoing need for nutritional assistance (Dubowitz, 2021; Dubowitz et al., 2023).

Access to and Experience with Health Care Services

Health Care Access and Use

Insurance is an important facilitator of access to health care. Nearly all (97.1 percent) of respondents reported having some form of health insurance coverage (see Table 2.8). The different types of coverage are not mutually exclusive. For example, a respondent may have both employer provided health insurance and Medicare. About half of respondents (47.9 percent) had employer provided insurance, 31.0 percent had TRICARE (the uniformed services health

TABLE 2.8

Rates of Insurance Coverage and Access to Health Care Services

Health Insurance	Percentage	95% CI LL	95% CI UL
Any health insurance	97.1	96.1	98.2
Source of health insurance[a]			
Employer provided	47.9	44.6	51.1
Direct purchase	2.8	1.7	3.8
Medicare	7.5	6.1	9.0
Medicaid	5.3	3.7	6.9
TRICARE	31.0	28.0	34.0
Any other type of plan	2.9	1.8	3.9
Have usual source of care	70.0	67.0	73.0
Access to health care services through VA	76.5	73.8	79.2
Those with access that received care at VA in past year	65.6	62.0	69.2
Those with access that received care in the community (paid for by VA) in past year	24.9	21.7	28.5

NOTE: LL = lower limit; UL = upper limit.

[a] Sources of insurance are not mutually exclusive.

care program), and 7.5 percent had Medicare. Approximately 70 percent reported having a usual source of care, a common marker of better access. This is the same as or lower than estimates for the general adult population, where estimates range from approximately 70 percent to 90 percent of the population reporting having a usual source of care (Agency for Healthcare Research and Quality, 2021; Peterson-KFF Health System Tracker, 2022). It is somewhat lower than nationally representative estimates for U.S. veterans aged 19 to 64 with approximately 78 percent reporting having a usual source of care (Bernard and Selden, 2016).

About three-quarters of respondents reported being able to access health care through VA. Among those, in the past year, 65.6 percent received care at a VA facility and 24.9 percent received care in the community that was paid for by VA.

When asked about their preferences on where to receive care if cost was not an issue, the majority of respondents (61 percent) preferred to see a community provider, with 46 percent (95-percent CI: 42.8–49.3) preferring one that is not associated with the military or VA and 15 percent (95-percent CI: 12.4–16.8) preferring a community provider that is. About one-third would prefer to receive treatment in a VA facility (see Figure 2.3). While not directly comparable, it is interesting to note that the proportion preferring community providers is higher than the 46 percent of respondents in 2010 who reported a preference for receiving mental health treatment from a civilian provider rather than VA.

Among those that reported a preference for a community provider (whether or not they were affiliated with the military or VA), easier access in the community was the most common

FIGURE 2.3

Preferences for Where to Receive Health Care Services

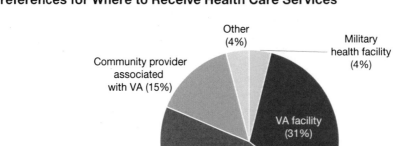

reason (48.5 percent; 95-percent CI: 44.4–52.6) for that preference (see Figure 2.4). Other common reasons respondents stated include the belief that the quality of care was better from a community provider (43.9 percent; 95-percent CI: 39.8–47.9) and the desire not to disrupt an already established relationship with a community provider (39.5 percent; 95-percent CI: 35.6–43.5). The least common reason, though still reported by about 20 percent [95-percent CI: 17.2–24.1], was due to a prior bad experience with VA.

Because the preference for community providers and the reasons for that preference may vary across veteran demographics, we looked at responses across age, gender, and rural/urban status. Younger veterans (under age 35) were more likely than older veterans to report a preference for community providers (65.7 percent vs. 55.1 percent) (see Table 2.9). Among those reporting a preference for community providers, older veterans were more likely than younger veterans to report an established relationship with a provider (46.5 percent vs. 30.0 percent) and easier access (53.2 percent vs. 42.0 percent) as reasons for that preference. No other differences across age were statistically significant.

Given differences in the availability of health care services at VA and in the community between urban and rural settings, we explored whether there were differences in preferences for community care. No differences were found between those currently residing in urban and rural areas (see Table 2.10).

Finally, because the number of women veterans is growing quickly and their health care needs and preferences may differ from men's, we looked at differences in preferences for community care between men and women veterans. There was no difference in the proportion between men and women (59.1 percent vs. 59.7 percent, $p = 0.897$) reporting a preference for community providers. The most commonly reported reasons for this preference among both men and women were perceived higher quality and easier access to care. In general, women were less likely to report any of the reasons than men, but most differences were not statistically significant (see Table 2.11).

FIGURE 2.4

Reasons for Preferring to Get Care from a Community Provider (among those with that preference; unweighted *n* = 677)

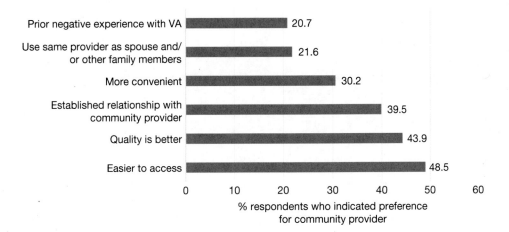

TABLE 2.9

Preferences for Where to Receive Health Care Services by Age

	Younger Veterans[a] (unweighted *n* = 383)			Older Veterans[b] (unweighted *n* = 737)			
	Percentage	95% CI LL	95% CI UL	Percentage	95% CI LL	95% CI UL	*p*-value[c]
Prefer care from a community provider	65.7	60.6	70.8	55.1	51.1	59.1	**0.001**
Reasons for preferring care from community providers (among those with that preference)							
Quality is better	41.6	35.0	48.1	45.3	40.3	50.4	0.365
Established relationship with community provider	30.0	24.0	35.9	46.5	41.4	51.5	**0.000**
Easier to access	42.0	35.4	48.6	53.2	48.1	58.2	**0.008**
More convenient	31.2	25.1	37.4	29.3	24.5	34.1	0.624
Use same provider as spouse and/ or other family members	18.5	13.3	23.7	24.0	19.4	28.7	0.120
Prior bad experience with VA care	23.9	17.8	29.9	18.2	14.3	22.0	0.122

NOTE: Bolded *p*-values are significant at the 5-percent level. LL = lower limit; UL = upper limit.

[a] Younger veterans defined as individuals aged 34 or younger.

[b] Older veterans defined as individuals aged 35 and above.

[c] *p*-value is from a chi-squared test of differences in the estimated proportion of younger and older veterans.

TABLE 2.10

Preferences for Where to Receive Health Care Services by Geography

	Live in urban[a] area (unweighted n = 977)			Live in rural[b] area (unweighted n = 146)			
	Percentage	95% CI LL	95% CI UL	Percentage	95% CI LL	95% CI UL	p-value[c]
Prefer care from a community provider	59.0	55.8	62.2	60.6	49.8	71.4	0.776
Reasons for preferring to get care from a community provider (among those with that preference)							
Quality is better	43.3	39.2	47.5	46.9	33.9	59.8	0.555
Established relationship with community provider	40.6	36.5	44.7	34.3	22.0	46.5	0.221
Easier to access	46.9	42.7	51.1	56.8	43.8	69.8	0.093
More convenient	28.9	25.1	32.7	37.0	24.3	49.7	0.169
Use same provider as spouse and/ or other family members	20.3	17.0	23.6	28.4	15.7	41.1	0.060
Prior bad experience with VA care	19.9	16.4	23.3	25.0	13.1	36.9	0.341

NOTE: LL = lower limit; UL = upper limit.

[a] Urban defined as residing in an MSA.

[b] Rural defined as not living in an MSA.

[c] p-value is from a chi-squared test of differences in the estimated proportion of respondents in urban and rural areas.

Use of Mental Health Care

About one-third of respondents (31.3 percent) reported visiting a doctor at least once for a mental health problem during the past year (see Table 2.12). This is somewhat higher than the 24 percent reported in the 2010 study (Farmer et al., 2011). Of those who had a mental health visit, 92 percent had at least one visit with a mental health specialist and 36.1 percent had at least one mental health visit with a regular medical doctor or primary care physician. To provide a sense of whether people with a demonstrated need for care were accessing services at higher rates, we looked at the use of mental health care among veterans who had a probable mental health diagnosis or reported suicidal ideation. Among veterans with some demonstrated need, the proportion having a mental health visit to a doctor was approximately double that of the full sample (see Figure 2.5). While the rate is higher in this group, still about 40 percent of those with a probable diagnosis or suicidal ideation did not report having a mental health visit in the past year.

TABLE 2.11

Preferences for Where to Receive Health Care Services by Gender

	Men (unweighted $n = 968$)			Women (unweighted $n = 147$)			
	Percentage	95% CI LL	95% CI UL	Percentage	95% CI LL	95% CI UL	p-value[a]
Prefer care from a community provider	59.1	55.7	62.6	59.7	50.9	68.6	0.897
Reasons for preferring care from community providers							
Quality is better	44.2	39.8	48.6	40.3	29.4	51.1	0.511
Established relationship with community provider	40.9	36.6	45.2	33.0	22.5	43.4	0.167
Easier to access	50.4	46.0	54.8	35.1	24.6	45.7	**0.009**
More convenient	30.4	26.3	34.5	29.3	19.3	39.3	0.841
Use same provider as spouse and/ or other family members	24.0	20.1	27.9	6.7	1.4	12.0	**0.000**
Prior bad experience with VA care	19.9	16.2	23.5	23.7	14.2	33.2	0.464

NOTE: Bolded p-values are significant at the 5-percent level. LL = lower limit; UL = upper limit.

[a] p-value is from a chi-squared test of differences in the estimated proportion of male and female.

TABLE 2.12

Past Year Mental Health Service Use Among Recently Separated Veterans

	All Respondents		
	Percentage	95% CI LL	95% CI UL
Any mental health visit	31.3	28.2	34.4
Nonspecialist doctor	36.1	29.9	42.5
Mental health specialist	92.0	89.0	94.9
Mental health treatment desired but not obtained	21.0	18.4	23.6

NOTE: LL = lower limit; UL = upper limit.

FIGURE 2.5

Proportion of Recently Separated Veterans with Probable Depression, Probable PTSD, and Suicidal Ideation That Reported Any Past Year Mental Health Visit

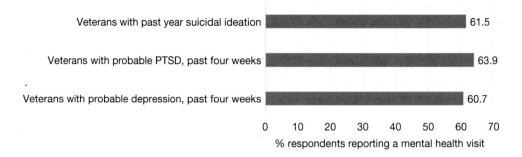

Unmet Need for Care

While nearly all respondents had some type of health insurance coverage, this did not ensure access to needed health care services. There is still substantial unmet need for both physical and mental health care among respondents. Fifteen percent (95-percent CI: 13.2–18.1) of respondents indicated that they had a need for physical health care services in the past year but did not get that care. This does not necessarily mean that these individuals did not receive any care, rather that they received less care than they felt was needed. The proportion with unmet need is somewhat higher than the 8.4 percent that was estimated for a nationally representative sample of veterans (Cohen and Boersma, 2023). Even more, 21.0 percent (95-percent CI: 18.4–23.6) reported an unmet need for mental health care in the past year, which is very similar to the 20 percent reported in the 2010 study (Farmer et al., 2011). Among veterans with a likely need for mental health services, the rate is much higher. For veterans with suicidal ideation in the past year, the proportion with unmet need for mental health care jumped to 43.4 percent, and for those with a probable mental health diagnosis (either depression or PTSD) the proportion with an unmet need was 38.9 percent.

For physical health care, the most common logistical barriers that respondents with unmet need noted were that services were not easily accessible (55.4 percent, 95-percent CI 47.0–63.8) and that the respondent lacked the supports (34.5 percent, 95-percent CI 26.5–42.5), such as child care or transportation, that would enable them to get care (see Figure 2.6). For respondents with unmet mental health needs, the logistical barriers were not endorsed by as many as among those with unmet physical health needs, but services not being easily accessible was still the most common barrier cited (30.7 percent, 95-percent CI 24.2–37.1). Some respondents additionally provided free text responses about other barriers they faced. In many cases, respondents used this as an opportunity to provide specific examples of types of barriers that were asked about. Many free text responses related to ways in which services were not easily accessible or unaffordable. The free text responses did, however, point to one additional category of barriers that people faced: a lack of motivation to seek care. We provide examples of specific responses in each of these categories in Figure 2.7.

FIGURE 2.6

Logistical Barriers Among Recently Separated Veterans Who Desire Physical Health Care (unweighted $n = 161$) and Mental Health Care (unweighted $n = 221$)

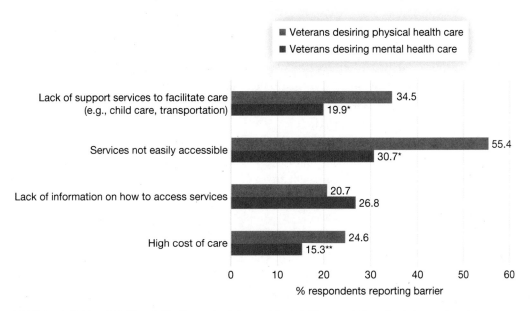

NOTE: $*p < 0.05$, $**p < 0.01$, $***p < 0.001$. The p-value is from an F-test of differences in the estimated proportion of respondents with unmet physical health and mental health needs reporting each logistical barrier.

FIGURE 2.7

Examples of Recently Separated Veterans' Free Text Responses About Barriers to Getting Needed Physical Health Care

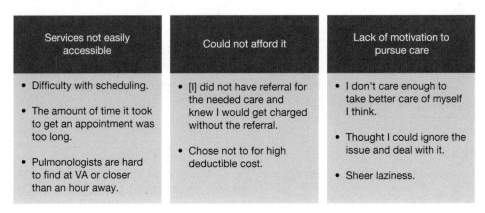

Respondents with unmet mental health care needs were additionally asked about how institutional and cultural barriers and their own beliefs about treatment affected their decision to seek care (see Table 2.13). The perceived stigma around mental health care was a big barrier for respondents. About one-quarter of respondents with unmet mental health needs said seeking care could harm their career and that they had concerns about what others would think if they sought care. This marks an improvement from the prior study where 33 percent reported that they felt seeking care could harm their career (Farmer et al., 2011). In addition, many respondents (38.8 percent) believed mental health treatment is ineffective and chose not to seek care. This is substantially higher than the 11 percent who reported this in the prior study (Farmer et al., 2011).

Respondents who had unmet mental health needs provided free text responses about other barriers that they faced in getting care. As with physical health care, many respondents used the opportunity to share specific examples of the types of barriers asked about, including services not being easily accessible and not having the supports needed to access services. For example, one respondent reported, "[I] could hardly make time to do the research on who I could see, let alone schedule an appointment. Work and family life are very busy." Numerous respondents reported prior negative experiences with mental health care providers as a reason for not seeking needed care. For example, one respondent said, "The therapist dismissed my concerns, so I stopped going," and another reported not getting care because "[I was] told that I didn't need the level of care I was seeking."

Given the potential effect of deployment on mental and physical health outcomes, we looked at differences between those with no combat deployments and those with at least one. When comparing health status and unmet health care needs of veterans with and without combat deployments, mental health disparities emerged while physical health and unmet need remained relatively consistent across groups (see Table 2.14). Veterans in the sample with combat exposure reported significantly lower rates of probable depression and higher rates of probable PTSD than veterans without deployments.

TABLE 2.13

Reasons for Not Seeking Mental Health Care Among Recently Separated Veterans Who Desire It (n = 221)

Reason	Percentage	95% CI LL	95% CI UL
Institutional and Cultural			
Professional help could harm veteran's career	26.4	20.2	32.6
Concerns about what others would think	27.2	20.9	33.5
Beliefs about Treatment			
Perceived ineffectiveness of mental health treatment	38.8	32.0	45.7
Concerns related to side effects of psychiatric medications	18.5	13.1	23.9

NOTE: LL = lower limit; UL = upper limit.

TABLE 2.14

Mental and Physical Health Status and Service Use by Combat Deployment Status

Mental or Physical Health Characteristic	Veterans with at Least One Combat Deployment (unweighted n = 698)			Veterans with no Combat Deployments (unweighted n = 425)			p-value
	Percentage or mean	95% CI LL	95% CI UL	Percentage or mean	95% CI LL	95% CI UL	
Mental health conditions							
Probable depression	21.8	18.5	25.2	28.6	23.4	33.9	**0.020**
Probable PTSD	28.7	24.7	32.6	20.9	15.9	25.8	**0.044**
Physical health status							
Physical functioning score (mean)	77.7	75.8	79.6	76.8	73.4	80.3	0.663
Role limitations score (mean)	71.1	68.5	73.6	71.5	67.4	75.6	0.870
Excellent or very good health	40.3	36.4	44.2	38.6	33.6	43.6	0.538
Unmet need for care in last year							
Physical health care	15.5	12.5	18.5	15.9	11.7	20.0	0.669
Mental health care	20.7	17.4	24.0	21.5	17.3	25.8	0.750

NOTE: p-value is for a chi-squared test of the difference in proportion between those with combat exposure and those without. Bolded p-values are significant at the 5-percent level. LL = lower limit; UL = upper limit.

Average physical functioning and role limitations scores, and the proportions reporting "excellent or very good" health status, were consistent between veterans with and without combat deployments. This finding is inconsistent with previous research suggesting increased risk for physical health conditions associated with combat deployments (Teplova et al., 2022). Of note, items included on the SF-36 measure used in the present study captured veterans' physical abilities as they relate to occupational and daily living tasks (e.g., climbing stairs, bathing oneself, performing work-related activities). Therefore, while the level of functional impairment appears to be consistent across respondents with and without deployments, any differences in the prevalence rates of specific physical health conditions that have been associated with combat deployment (e.g., asthma, headache, hearing loss, pain) remain unknown.

No significant differences in rates of perceived unmet needs for mental and physical health care were found across the two groups, highlighting that a significant proportion of recently separated veterans, regardless of combat exposure, have experienced difficulties accessing needed physical and mental health services. Rates of unmet need for physical health care (15.5–15.9 percent) were lower than rates of unmet need for mental health care (20.7–21.5 percent), suggesting that recently separated veterans living in New York may have particular difficulty accessing needed mental health services.

Experiences of Care

Respondents that received care in a VA facility and those that received care through VA's community care network in the past year were asked about their experiences with that care. Figures 2.8 through 2.10 present information on those experiences and how they differed between VA facilities and community providers. Overall, experiences in both settings were generally positive.

Among respondents receiving care in a VA facility, 87.9 percent (95-percent CI: 84.7–91.2) reported that the staff were welcoming and helpful always or most of the time. About three-quarters reported that appointments were available on convenient days and times always or most of the time (74.6 percent, 95-percent CI: 70.5–78.6). They were also generally satisfied or very satisfied with elements of their VA care. About 90 percent of respondents reported being satisfied with the respect shown to them by their care team (88.1 percent, 95-percent CI: 84.9–91.3) and with the way their privacy was protected (91.0 percent, 95-percent CI: 88.4–93.5). Upward of 80 percent indicated being satisfied with how clearly the provider explained their health care options and choices (84.3 percent, 95-percent CI: 80.9–87.8) and how they provided opportunities for the respondent to participate in decisions about care (82.0 percent, 95-percent CI: 78.3–85.8). Among the experiences considered, respondents were least satisfied with their ability to get referrals for specialist care or special equipment (73.7 percent reporting being satisfied or very satisfied, 95-percent CI: 69.6–77.7).

Among respondents receiving care through a VA community care network, about 90 percent reported that the staff were welcoming and helpful (90.6 percent, 95-percent CI: 86.0–95.1) and that it was easy to get to their appointment most of or all the time (89.4 percent, 95-percent CI: 84.5–94.2). Eighty-two percent reported that most of or all the time they could get appointments within a reasonable time frame (82.3 percent, 95-percent CI: 76.2–88.4)

FIGURE 2.8

Recently Separated Veterans' Experiences of Care in Past Year, by Site of Service

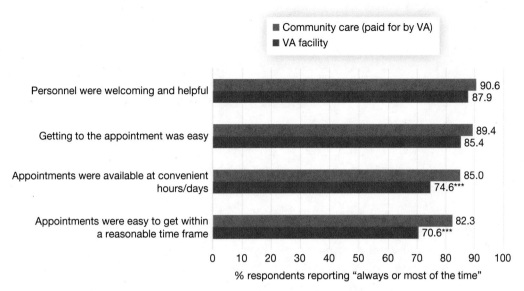

Legend:
- ■ Community care (paid for by VA)
- ■ VA facility

Personnel were welcoming and helpful — 90.6 / 87.9

Getting to the appointment was easy — 89.4 / 85.4

Appointments were available at convenient hours/days — 85.0 / 74.6***

Appointments were easy to get within a reasonable time frame — 82.3 / 70.6***

X-axis: 0 10 20 30 40 50 60 70 80 90 100
% respondents reporting "always or most of the time"

NOTE: $*p<0.05$, $**p<0.01$, $***p<0.001$. The p-value is from an F-test of differences in the estimated proportion of respondents receiving care at a VA facility or community care reporting that response option.

FIGURE 2.9

Recently Separated Veterans' Satisfaction with Care in Past Year, by Site of Service

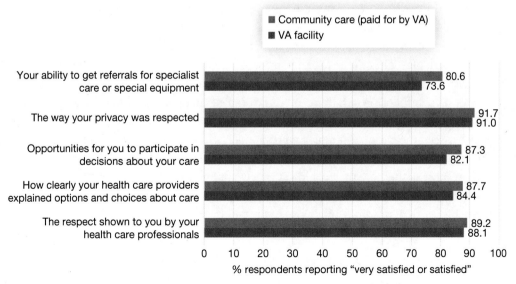

Legend:
- ■ Community care (paid for by VA)
- ■ VA facility

Your ability to get referrals for specialist care or special equipment — 80.6 / 73.6

The way your privacy was respected — 91.7 / 91.0

Opportunities for you to participate in decisions about your care — 87.3 / 82.1

How clearly your health care providers explained options and choices about care — 87.7 / 84.4

The respect shown to you by your health care professionals — 89.2 / 88.1

X-axis: 0 10 20 30 40 50 60 70 80 90 100
% respondents reporting "very satisfied or satisfied"

NOTE: $*p<0.05$, $**p<0.01$, $***p<0.001$. The p-value is from an F-test of differences in the estimated proportion of respondents receiving care at a VA facility or community care reporting that response option.

FIGURE 2.10

Recently Separated Veterans' Perceptions of Military Cultural Competence, by Site of Service

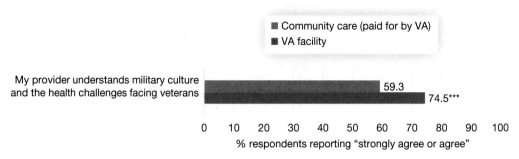

NOTE: $*p<0.05$, $**p<0.01$, $***p<0.001$. The p-value is from an F-test of differences in the estimated proportion of respondents receiving care at a VA facility or community care reporting that response option.

and 85.0 percent (95-percent CI: 79.6–90.4) reported they were able to get appointments at convenient days and times. Respondents receiving care in the community were generally satisfied, with over 80 percent of respondents reporting being satisfied or very satisfied with all aspects of care they were asked about.

The primary differences found between veterans' experiences of care at a VA facility versus through VA's community care network related to access. Those receiving care in the community were more likely to indicate being able to get appointments within a reasonable time frame most of or all the time (82.3 percent for community care vs. 70.6 for VA care) and at times that were convenient for them (85.0 percent for community care vs. 74.5 percent for VA care). In contrast, respondents receiving VA care were much more likely than those receiving community care to agree or strongly agree that their usual provider understands military culture and the health challenges facing veterans (74.5 percent for VA care vs. 59.3 percent for community care). No other differences were statistically significant.

The pattern of results related to experiences of care for recently separated veterans in New York is very similar to what was found in a national sample of VA health care enrollees in 2022, in which enrollees generally reported favorable experiences and satisfaction with their care at both VA facilities and with community care providers (VA, 2022). The primary difference between the national sample and respondents in this sample relates to timely access. In the national sample of VA enrollees who received care at a VA facility, 87 percent reported that all or most of the time they could get timely appointments compared with 70.5 percent in this sample of veterans (VA, 2022). This suggests that wait times for appointments in New York are higher than in some other parts of the country.

Use of Other Services for Veterans

Respondents were asked about different types of services that are available to veterans; whether or not they had ever used these services; and, regardless of use, whether they would find them helpful. For most types of services, the proportion of respondents who thought such a service would be helpful was larger than the proportion who reported having used the benefit (see Figure 2.11). The biggest discrepancies between perceived utility and actual use of benefits were reported for reduced costs of health insurance for self or family (48.2 percent helpful vs. 11.2 percent used), housing assistance or loans (45.8 percent helpful vs. 18.9 percent used), and job training (33.8 percent helpful vs. 9.9 percent used). Receiving health care at VA was one exception where 62.8 percent of respondents said they had used that benefit, but

FIGURE 2.11

Benefits and Services Ever Used and Perceived as Helpful by Recently Separated Veterans

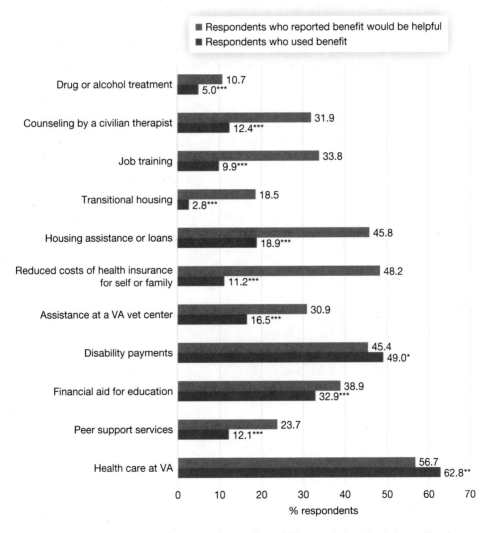

NOTE: *$p < 0.05$, **$p < 0.01$, ***$p < 0.001$. The p-value is from an F-test of differences in the estimated proportion of respondents reporting use of the service and the proportion reporting that the benefit would be useful.

only 56.6 percent reported they thought it would be helpful. Disability payments was the other exception where 49.0 percent reported using the benefit and 45.4 percent reported that it would be helpful. Following VA care and disability payments, the most frequently used benefits were financial aid for education (32.9 percent, 95-percent CI: 29.8–36.0), housing assistance or loans (18.9 percent, 95-percent CI: 16.3–21.5), and assistance at a VA vet center (16.5 percent, 95-percent CI: 13.9–19.2). The least commonly used benefits by veterans in the sample were transitional housing (2.8 percent, 95-percent CI: 1.4–4.1) and drug or alcohol treatment (5.0 percent, 95-percent CI: 3.2–6.9).

The benefits most commonly identified as helpful by respondents included VA health care (56.6 percent, 95-percent CI: 53.4–59.9), reduced cost of health insurance for self or family (48.2 percent, 95-percent CI: 45.0–51.5), and housing assistance or loans (45.8 percent, 95-percent CI: 42.5–49.0). About one-third of respondents thought job training, financial aid for education, and counseling from a therapist would be helpful. The benefit that the fewest respondents thought would be helpful was drug or alcohol treatment (10.7 percent, 95-percent CI: 8.4–12.9). Compared with the 2010 study, fewer veterans in the current sample reported they thought these benefits would be helpful (Farmer et al., 2011).

Finally, we asked veterans about their understanding of what benefits were available to them and their knowledge of where they can go to get answers to questions about their benefits. About one-quarter of respondents agreed or strongly agreed that they did know what benefits were available to them (24.0 percent, 95-percent CI: 21.2–26.8) and where to get answers about those benefits (25.4 percent, 95-percent CI: 22.6–28.2). This suggests that many veterans were unsure of what types of benefits they could potentially access and how to get information about those benefits, implying a need for continued and expanded outreach to veterans about the benefits they are eligible for.

CHAPTER 3

Implications and Recommendations

The results of this survey indicate that recently separated veterans in New York currently face a number of mental and physical health challenges. Approximately a quarter of respondents screened positive for probable depression and probable PTSD and about 9 percent reported suicidal thoughts. The veterans in this sample had a high rate of self-reported disability and experienced poor self-reported physical health, regardless of whether they experienced a combat deployment, compared with the general population norm for the same age and gender distribution. These findings point to poorer physical health outcomes for *all* recently separated veterans, not only those with combat deployments or military-related disabilities (Schnittker, 2018).

While nearly all respondents had some form of health insurance, that did not necessarily translate into adequate access to mental and physical health care. Between 15 and 20 percent of veterans reported having needs for mental or physical care in the past year and not having them met. The rate of unmet need for mental health care was even higher (38.8 percent) among veterans in the sample with a probable mental health diagnosis. The primary barriers to getting needed physical and mental health care that were noted were related to a lack of support services that would facilitate access, such as transportation assistance and child care, and to services being offered in inconvenient locations or times. Regarding additional unmet needs, a significant proportion of respondents (26 percent) reported having experienced food insecurity within the past year.

Among those who accessed health care services either at a VA facility or through VA's community care network, the experiences of and satisfaction with the care they received were generally very positive. Despite this positive experience, many veterans (47 percent) indicated that if they could get care anywhere free of charge, they would prefer to get that care from a community provider that is not associated with the military or VA. The most common reasons for this preference were related to perceptions of easier access and better quality of care.

Recently separated veterans in New York reported accessing a range of benefits and services (e.g., housing assistance or loans, financial aid for education). However, in nearly all cases the proportion of respondents that thought a given benefit would be useful was larger than the proportion who had used that benefit. This could reflect an unmet need for services for some respondents; for others it may reflect that they view the benefit as useful in general but do not have a need for it themselves at this time. Additionally, only a quarter of respondents reported understanding which benefits they were eligible for.

Comparison with 2010 Needs Assessment of Veterans Living in New York

RAND used the same data source and survey design as the 2010 needs assessment of veterans in New York (Farmer et al., 2011) to provide insights on the health and well-being of recently separated veterans and their access to, use of, and perceptions of services. The 2010 and 2024 samples, however, vary in critical ways that limit direct comparisons made between the two studies. The prior study focused on recently discharged veterans who had deployed at least once to either OIF or OEF. For the current study, we did not require that a veteran had been deployed to be eligible for inclusion. In fact, approximately 40 percent of the current sample reported no deployments during their time in the military. More generally, the population of veterans in New York has changed over time and become more diverse (see Figure 3.1). The current sample of veterans is older (38.6 percent vs. 54 percent under age 35), more diverse in terms or race and gender (62 percent vs. 73 percent White; 14.7 percent vs. 11 percent female), and more educated (49.7 percent vs. 33 percent with a college degree or higher) than those included in the prior study. At the same time, the samples are similar across other dimensions including employment (70.5 percent vs. 72 percent currently employed either full- or part-time) and rank at time of separation (80 percent vs. 82 percent enlisted personnel).

On the key measures of health and well-being that are common across studies, the current cohort of veterans reported more mental and physical health problems than were found in the prior study. Approximately one-quarter of respondents screened positive for depression (24.6 percent) and PTSD (25.5 percent) compared with 16 percent for each condition in the prior study. This may reflect the upward trend in the prevalence of mental health problems, including mood disorder symptoms and suicide-related outcomes, seen nationwide among adults since 2010, which has further increased since the beginning of the COVID-19 pandemic in 2020 (Goodwin et al., 2022; Twenge et al., 2019). The current cohort of veterans reported substantially more disability and poorer physical health. The proportion of veterans with a service-connected disability rating was 62.8 percent in the current sample compared with 31 percent in 2010. Among those with a disability rating, the average percentage disability was also much higher (68.5 percent vs. 38 percent). The change since 2010 is consistent with the increase in the proportion of veterans with a service-connected disability from about 10 percent in 2000 to about 25 percent in 2018 (VA, 2019) and may reflect both greater disability and changes in disability definitions and policy over time. The current sample also scored lower on the scales assessing physical functioning and role limitations than the veterans in the prior study, but the scores compared with the age- and sex-adjusted norms for the general population were similar at about 0.2 to 0.3 standard deviations below the norm.

Consistent with the higher rate of mental health problems observed in the current cohort of veterans, a larger proportion of respondents reported using mental health services in the prior year than did so in the 2010 study (31.3 percent vs. 24 percent). However, the proportion reporting an unmet need for mental health services did not significantly change between the two samples (21 percent vs. 20 percent). While the rate is similar, the reported barriers to

FIGURE 3.1

Cohorts of Recently Separated Veterans in New York: 2010 Versus 2024

DEMOGRAPHICS

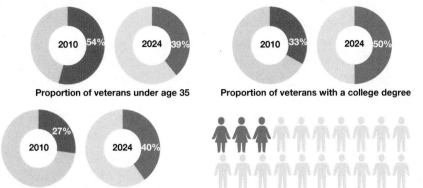

Proportion of veterans under age 35

2010 54% 2024 39%

Proportion of veterans with a college degree

2010 33% 2024 50%

Proportion of veterans who were from racial or ethnic minority backgrounds

2010 27% 2024 40%

Compared to 11% in 2010, 15% of the 2023 sample were women

PHYSICAL AND MENTAL HEALTH CHARACTERISTICS

Veterans' overall physical functioning scores remained relatively consistent across the two cohorts (below average physical health relative to nonveterans). However, rates of disability and mental health concerns were higher in 2023.

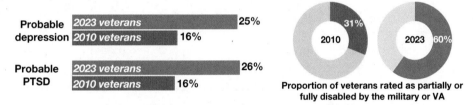

Probable depression
- 2023 veterans: 25%
- 2010 veterans: 16%

Probable PTSD
- 2023 veterans: 26%
- 2010 veterans: 16%

2010 31% 2023 60%

Proportion of veterans rated as partially or fully disabled by the military or VA

USE OF MENTAL HEALTH SERVICES

Proportion of veterans who use mental health services
- 2023 veterans: 32%
- 2010 veterans: 24%

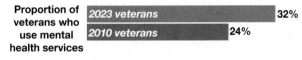

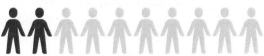

In both cohorts, 2 in 10 veterans reported not receiving needed mental health services.

Among veterans with unmet mental health needs, the proportion reporting certain reasons for not accessing care increased, while it decreased for other reasons.

↑ **Not knowing where to find right services.**
Reported by 27% in 2023 vs. 12% in 2010

↑ **Believe mental health care will not be effective.**
Reported by 39% in 2023 vs. 11% in 2010

↓ **Concerns seeking care will harm their career.**
Reported by 27% in 2023 vs. 33% in 2010

↓ **Concerns about side effects associated with medications.**
Reported by 19% in 2023 vs. 35% in 2010

getting needed mental health services are somewhat different. In the current sample, veterans with unmet mental health needs were more likely than those in the prior study to report not knowing how to find the right services (26.8 percent vs. 12 percent) and believing that the care would not be effective (38.8 percent vs. 11 percent). Veterans in the current study were less likely to report concerns that seeking care could harm their career (26.4 percent vs. 33 percent) and concerns about side effects associated with psychiatric medications (18.5 percent vs. 35 percent).

Comparing the proportion of veterans using different types of benefits across the two studies, the results showed that the use rate was higher for some benefits and lower for others. The current cohort of veterans was more likely to report use of disability payments (49 percent vs. 29 percent), housing assistance or loans (18.9 percent vs. 9 percent), and job training (9.9 percent vs. 6 percent), and they were less likely to report use of assistance at a VA vet center (16.5 percent vs. 28 percent). The perceived usefulness of benefits, regardless of whether they had been used, however, decreased for nearly all categories from what was reported by veterans in 2010. The largest decreases were seen for financial aid for education (38.8 percent vs. 61 percent reporting it would be useful) and assistance at a VA vet center (30.8 percent vs. 53 percent reporting it would be useful).

Recommendations for Policy and Programs

The results from this survey point to several potential policy and programmatic changes that could improve services for veterans in New York.

Enhance access to and use of mental health services. Survey results indicate high rates of probable depression, probable PTSD, and suicide ideation among recently separated veterans. There is also substantial unmet need for mental health care. Given these findings, programs and policies should focus on increasing access to and use of mental health services. Given the preference for and use of community care, increasing the number of mental health professionals trained to work with veterans and integrating mental health services into primary care settings could be an impactful strategy for connecting more veterans with mental health care. To improve uptake of services, it will also be important to address veterans' perceptions around the effectiveness of mental health care and concerns about stigma associated with seeking care, possibly through innovative social marketing and public awareness campaigns that include service members who are just beginning their transition out of military service. Additionally, given the high rate of mental health care utilization among veterans with suicidal ideation in the sample, it is critical that evidence-based suicide prevention strategies (e.g., screening, lethal means counseling, safety planning) be systematically integrated into mental health care settings.

Continue to prioritize veteran-specific suicide prevention programs. Rates of past year suicidal ideation among recently separated veterans in New York were over twice as high as recent estimates from the general adult population in New York. Additionally, nearly half

(43 percent) of veterans with past-year suicidal ideation reported not obtaining needed mental health treatment (compared with 21 percent of all respondents). As these numbers demonstrate, continued dedication to veteran suicide prevention efforts is essential. Resources should be put toward creating more comprehensive, timely, and high-quality data infrastructure that captures suicide outcomes of veterans across New York state (overall and among demographic subgroups) and integrates data from both VA and community-based organizations. Such data can be used to support tailoring and implementation of evidence-based suicide prevention strategies to meet veterans' unique needs. As previous research shows, veterans who die by suicide are more likely to use firearms than civilians (Ramchand, 2021). The survey results illustrate that a significant proportion (over 40 percent) of recently separated veterans in New York have firearms in their homes, many of which are stored loaded (27 percent) or unlocked (37 percent). Continued investment in the implementation and evaluation of evidence-based gun safety counseling interventions (e.g., the Counseling on Access to Lethal Means [CALM] model) may be a key suicide prevention strategy for this group. Additionally, to address the unmet mental health needs of New York veterans at risk for suicide, a multipronged approach is needed. Additional priority prevention strategies may include but are not limited to research on barriers to mental health care among high-risk veterans, public education campaigns to increase awareness of existing services (e.g., Veterans Crisis Line), integration of suicide prevention into routine care settings (e.g., screening in primary care), and the expansion and evaluation of existing veteran-specific crisis intervention services (e.g., peer support programs).

Support veterans' ability to access both VA-based and community-based health care services. Recently separated New York veterans' preferences for where to receive health care varied, with about one-third preferring VA facilities and about two-thirds preferring community providers. Maintaining choice and access to the different care settings is needed to meet the diverse needs of veterans across New York state. Veterans that expressed a preference for receiving health care from a provider in the community instead of a provider at a VA facility believed they had better access and received higher-quality care in the community. Policies and programs should support veterans' ability to choose community-based health care providers and help them to identify and access high-quality services. At the same time, veterans noted that community-based health care providers were less likely to understand military culture and the special needs of veterans. As such, policies and programs could focus on ensuring that community providers have access to training and resources to help them meet the specific needs of veterans. This could include developing and disseminating training curricula around military cultural competence or standards of care for treating service-related conditions that are not as common in the general population. Strategies from implementation science will likely be needed to enhance uptake of training, in part because veterans may represent a small proportion of a community-based provider's patient population.

Address logistical barriers veterans face to accessing needed health care. Despite near universal health insurance coverage and high rates of VA facility utilization among recently separated veterans in New York, a significant proportion of veterans reported unmet health care needs and described multiple logistical barriers to accessing services (e.g., lack of transportation, child care, appointments at inconvenient days/times). This points to the importance of efforts to not only maintain insurance coverage for needed services but to also expand logistical supports (e.g., monetary assistance for transportation, evening and weekend hours for appointments) available to veterans to facilitate their ability to access and engage in treatment. To support veterans in accessing services and programs located near to them, veterans could be supported in using the Veterans Health Information Clearing House (New York State Department of Health, 2023) and the free NYS [New York State] Veterans mobile app (NYS Office of Information Technology Services, 2024). The app allows veterans to use location services to identify the address and contact information for nearby New York State Department of Veterans' Services field offices and related programs. Further, veterans can stay up-to-date with information regarding state and federal veterans' assistance programs and file claims for benefits directly via the app.

Improve and expand outreach and awareness about benefits and services, including those that address toxic exposures and food insecurity. Many veterans were unaware of the benefits available to them or did not perceive them as useful. This suggests a need to expand and improve outreach efforts to ensure veterans are informed about their eligibility for various benefits and services. Efforts to do so could involve partnerships with and among VA and community organizations, targeted information campaigns, and the use of technology to reach a broader audience. Given that nearly half of respondents believed they had a health condition related to toxic chemical exposure during military service, veterans in New York may benefit from targeted outreach on the relevant New York state veterans' services law that entitles eligible veterans and members of the reserves/National Guard to receive a health screening to test for exposure and subsequent treatment as indicated (see New York State Senate, 2023). Additionally, there is a pressing need for veteran-specific campaigns aimed at increasing awareness and utilization of food assistance programs among veterans and their families in New York. Researchers have identified state-level policies and programs that facilitate food-insecure veterans use of food assistance programs, including broad-based categorical eligibility for SNAP (i.e., increasing gross income limits for eligibility), streamlining SNAP and social security applications, and call centers (Dubowitz et al., 2023). Veterans should therefore be made aware of New York state's current broad-based categorical eligibility for SNAP, and eligible veterans should be supported in the process of applying for benefits. To supplement ongoing efforts inside VA that already are working to address veteran food insecurity (e.g., food insecurity screenings and on-site food pantries), specific outreach to food-insecure New York veterans not enrolled in VA is critical. It will also be important to understand more about how to make existing benefits more useful as well as about what additional benefits would be valued. This could be done through continued engagement with veterans, overall and among specific subgroups, to gather more detailed information about their needs, what they perceive to be useful and why, and any barriers they face. The expansion of existing veteran peer support and care coordination programs may also help veterans to navigate the complex landscape of available services throughout New York state and to address stigma related to use of benefits.

Consider the growing diversity of the veteran population when designing and implementing policies and programs. The increasing diversity among veterans in New York, including more veteran women, LGBTQ+ veterans (Grogan et al., 2020), and those from racial and ethnic minority backgrounds, indicates a need to ensure services are inclusive and culturally responsive. This could involve training for service providers on equity and cultural competency and developing programs that specifically address the unique challenges faced by these subgroups. Additionally, program administrators could evaluate and optimize such efforts through the ongoing assessment of patient experience and patient-centered outcomes and engagement in quality improvement efforts.

Limitations

This study is subject to several limitations. First, our sample was designed to be representative of veterans in New York who recently separated from the military, not the full population of veterans in New York. As such, we were unable to find appropriate external benchmarks for this population against which we could compare our sample to understand and account for potential nonresponse biases. There are some publicly available datasets that provide information on the veteran population, such as the CPS Veterans Supplement (see IPUMS CPS, undated), however, when looking at the data for New York, the sample size was too small and skewed toward older veterans to be useful for this purpose. Instead, we used urbanicity and proxies for age, gender, and race/ethnicity based on names and addresses for the full list we received and used that information to create nonresponse weights. Still, the sample looks different from the full population of veterans. Two key differences are that the current sample reported an average of nearly 15 years of service in the military and over 40 percent reported being retired from the military, which are both much higher than what is seen in the full population of veterans. Second, it is possible that some people who were not part of the eligible sample completed the survey. We used a variety of mechanisms to prevent this from occurring, including updating addresses using LexisNexis, asking directly as part of the questions screening for eligibility, and comparing contact information provided at the end of the survey to receive the gift card with the sampled person's name. Still, it is possible that some people who were not sampled completed the survey.

Third, the response rate to the survey was approximately 13 percent. While this is low overall, it is in the expected range compared with others conducted using letters with push-to-web for completing the survey (Parast et al., 2019; Sauermann and Roach, 2013). We used several methods to increase the response rate. To start, we tested several versions of fielding procedures in our pilot test to identify the best approach to balance response rates and costs. When fielding the survey, we sent multiple letters and email reminders and extended the time over which the survey was open.

Given the nature of the survey, veterans mainly responded to close-ended and multiple-choice response questions, so certain perspectives or answer types may not have been captured. Therefore, it could be beneficial to follow up these findings with in-depth qualitative interviews or focus groups with recently separated veterans living in New York. This qualitative data would provide a more in-depth understanding of veterans' diverse health needs, barriers to care, and patterns of service use that could elucidate additional factors affecting veterans' well-being and recommendations for policy and practice changes.

Conclusion

Despite these limitations, the survey results provide important information about the health and well-being of recently separated veterans living in New York. The results can be used to better understand this cohort of veterans' needs, the barriers they face in accessing services, and their experiences with VA health care. More importantly, they can inform changes in programs and policies to improve awareness of, access to, and use of needed services among veterans in New York.

Survey Methods

Sampling and Procedures

The data that served as the basis for our sample of veterans in New York state were obtained through a RONA from VA. Title 38 of the U.S. Code authorizes the Secretary of Veterans Affairs to release the names or addresses of former members of the Armed Forces to non-profit organizations when the purpose of the release is directly connected with the conduct of programs and the use of benefits covered by Title 38. Our request met the criteria as the information gathered through the survey can be used by veteran service organizations to help address service gaps and barriers to accessing benefits and services to which veterans are entitled and could result in veterans applying for and/or receiving one or more benefits provided under Title 38.

We requested names and addresses of individuals discharged from the military in the last five years who listed a home address in New York state at the time of discharge. We received 30,907 records through the RONA that we believe includes individuals who were discharged between January 2018 and January 2023. To prepare the data for sampling, we removed duplicate observations and those with missing address information. The remaining 30,194 records served as the basis for our sample.

We initially drew a random sample of 1,250 records for use in pilot testing different fielding approaches (replicate 1). We used two commercial databases, V12 and LexisNexis, to update and format mailing addresses and where available add email addresses. After updating addresses, we removed 492 records with addresses outside of New York, leaving 758 records. To have a sample of approximately 1,250 for the pilot test we pulled a second random sample of 811 records and used the same process to update addresses, append emails, and remove those with addresses outside New York (replicate 2). The combination of these two replicates yielded a sample of 1,237 records with addresses in New York to be fielded in the pilot test. For the main survey sample (replicate 3), we drew a random sample of 18,500 cases from the remaining records. Based on our experience with the pilot test, we chose to only use LexisNexis for address updates and email appends for the main sample. After updating addresses, cases with addresses outside of New York were excluded, resulting in 11,279 eligible cases for the main survey fielding.

Data collection occurred in two stages. We first pilot tested five survey fielding approaches to identify one that would ensure adequate response rate with the resources available. We randomized the sample across the five arms (approximately 250 in each). Each arm received two mailings, differing by content (letter, letter and hardcopy of survey) of the envelope and means of delivery (USPS, FedEx). Table A.1 shows the two mailings for each of the five arms. All letter mailings were push-to-web and included a generic QR code and survey URL for respondents to complete the survey by web and a unique PIN to allow the respondent to enter the survey. The second mailing for arms C, D, and E, included a hardcopy survey and were mailed either via USPS or FedEx. The hardcopy surveys were accompanied by a cover letter and business-reply envelope. For all arms, up to four email reminders with personalized links to the survey were sent to any respondent with an associated email. The pilot data collection took place in November and December 2023.

Based on the results of the pilot testing, we decided to field the main survey using USPS letters for both the first and second mailing (arm B). This approach was the least expensive per case and achieved a response rate that was similar to the others. Using the AAPOR Response Rate Calculator 4, the pilot survey across all arms achieved a 15.1 percent response rate (AAPOR, undated). For the main sample, a total of five email reminders distributed throughout the fielding period were sent to the cases with email. Data collection for the main sample took place in February and March 2024. The response rate from the 11,279 fielded in the main survey was 12.5 percent. Across both the pilot and the main survey, we offered respondents who completed the survey a $25 gift card to thank them for their time and input. Across the pilot and main survey fielding, we received 1,171 completed or partially completed surveys from eligible respondents, representing an overall response rate (again using the AAPOR Response Rate Calculator 4) of 12.7 percent.

All potential respondents were screened for eligibility at the beginning of the survey. We sought to verify residence in New York and veteran status. We asked each respondent whether he or she

1. currently lives in New York
2. has previously served in the military
3. is currently on active duty.

To be eligible, respondents had to answer "Yes" to questions 1 and 2 and "No" to question 3. We also asked the respondent to verify that they were the person to whom the letter or email was addressed. Respondents who are currently in the National Guard or reserves, but are not currently on active duty, are included in the sample. This group differs from others in the sample because they were still serving in some capacity and that continued connec-

TABLE A.1

Pilot Test Design

	Arm A	Arm B	Arm C	Arm D	Arm E
1st mailing	USPS letter	USPS letter	FedEx letter	USPS letter	USPS letter
2nd mailing	FedEx letter	USPS letter	USPS survey	USPS survey	FedEx survey

tion to the military may have affected the measures we assess. At the same time, to be in the sample frame (i.e., the list of names and addresses from VA), they must have separated from the military in the past five years and are likely eligible for some veteran benefits. We looked at how this group differs from others in their responses to questions about demographics, health status, and benefit use (see Table A.2). While there are differences in demographics and health status (e.g., the National Guard or reserves group is younger and healthier), many of those who report being in the National Guard or reserves do have access to (65.3 percent) and use health care services through VA. Among those with access, 26.0 percent received care at a VA facility and 5.8 percent received care through VA's community care network.

All survey materials used in this needs assessment were reviewed and approved by the RAND Human Subjects Protection Committee prior to data collection. All respondents gave written informed consent to participate. They were informed that their responses would be kept confidential and would not be shared with the military or VA.

Sample Weights

The utility of weighting for this survey is unclear since the sample frame defines an ambiguous population, veterans who were recently discharged from the military. As such, we were unable to find appropriate external benchmarks for this population against which we could compare our sample to understand and assess representativeness. There are some publicly available datasets that provide information on the veteran population, such as the CPS Veterans Supplement (see IPUMS CPS, undated), however, when looking at the data for New York, the sample size was too small and skewed toward older veterans to be useful for this purpose. However, nonresponse adjustments still merit consideration as certain groups may be much less likely to respond than others, and systematic nonresponse may yield misleading survey findings.

Since the sample was selected from the sample frame using simple random sampling, no adjustment needed to be made for the survey design. However, to account for nonresponse, we used inverse probability weighting with a nonresponse model that accounts for characteristics that are observed for both respondents and nonrespondents. These characteristics are highly limited since the information available for the entire sample frame includes only the veterans' name and address. However, the characteristics used in the nonresponse model include

1. a proxy for race (White, Black, Hispanic, other)
2. urbanicity (rural, urban)
3. a proxy for gender (female, male)
4. a proxy for age.

The proxy for race is determined using the Bayesian Improved Surname Geocoding (BISG) algorithm (Elliott et al., 2009), which gives the probability that an individual falls into each of the four race categories given their surname and address.

TABLE A.2

Selected Demographics, Health Status, and Benefit Use Characteristics by Whether Currently in the National Guard or Reserves

Characteristics	Not Currently in National Guard or Reserves (unweighted n = 1,006)			Currently in National Guard or Reserves (unweighted n = 116)			p-value
	Percentage or mean	95% CI LL	95% CI UL	Percentage or mean	95% CI LL	95% CI UL	
Demographics							
Age (mean)	42.7	41.8	43.6	37.4	35.9	39.0	**0.000**
Black	13.3	10.5	16.1	10.3	4.2	16.4	0.381
Hispanic	16.4	13.6	19.2	17.2	8.9	25.4	0.871
White	61.6	58.1	65.1	63.7	53.8	73.7	0.696
Other	8.4	6.7	10.2	8.8	2.1	15.5	0.920
Male	85.1	82.5	87.6	85.9	78.4	93.3	0.847
Physical and Mental Health							
Physical functioning score (mean)	76.3	74.4	78.2	86.1	81.8	90.3	**0.000**
Role limitations score (mean)	70.1	67.7	72.5	80.9	75.6	86.3	**0.000**
Probable depression	25.4	22.2	28.5	17.7	9.9	25.6	0.077
Probable PTSD	26.9	23.6	30.2	14.4	6.3	22.4	**0.005**
Health Care Access and Use							
Access to care through VA	77.8	75.0	80.5	65.3	56.0	74.6	**0.012**
Received care at VA facility	68.4	64.7	72.1	37.8	26.0	49.6	**0.000**
Received care in community paid for by VA	25.9	22.3	29.5	15.7	5.8	25.6	0.059

NOTE: p-value is for a chi-squared test of the difference in proportion between those in the National Guard or reserves and others. Bolded p-values are significant at the 5-percent level. LL = lower limit; UL = upper limit.

Urbanicity is determined by geocoding addresses and mapping them into MSAs. If an address is located in an MSA it was coded as urban.

The proxy for gender is determined by matching each veteran's first name to social security databases and then establishing the probability that individuals in the database with the respective first name are of a given gender. A similar approach is taken to determine the proxy for age.

An optimization algorithm is used to estimate the probability of response for individuals in the various demographic categories by using the estimated likelihood of each sampled veteran falling into the given categories.

The characteristics as described above were input into a logistic regression model where an indicator of response was used as the outcome. Cases that failed to provide sufficient information for analysis were treated as nonrespondents for this model and therefore were not given a weight. A respondent needed to provide useful information for at least 50 percent of the items for which they were eligible to receive a weight (approximately 50 respondents failed to do so). The sample used for analysis included 1,122 veterans. The weights are then set as the inverse of the predicted probabilities from this model.

Table A.3 below provides an indication of how well the proxies of the demographic characteristics performed. The first column of the table (labeled "Survey Responses") indicates what percentage of the survey respondents fall into the respective demographic categories

TABLE A.3

Performance of the Demographic Probabilities Used in Weighting and Estimated Response Weights

	Survey Responses	Aggregated Probabilities			Response Rate
		Respondents	Surveyed	All NY	
White	69.4%	71.4%	66.0%	65.1%	10.0%
Black	10.3%	9.3%	10.8%	11.7%	7.1%
Hispanic	11.4%	11.3%	15.7%	15.8%	5.4%
Other	8.9%	8.1%	7.5%	7.4%	10.2%
Rural	13.0%	13.1%	16.2%	20.7%	7.2%
Urban	87.0%	86.9%	83.8%	79.3%	9.3%
Male	86.8%	85.8%	84.3%	83.9%	9.2%
Female	13.2%	14.2%	15.7%	16.1%	7.8%
Mean age	43.77	43.41	41.74	41.45	
Younger: (0–33)	29.6%	29.8%	34.3%	35.2%	5.5%
Middle: (33–54)	44.5%	43.3%	42.9%	42.8%	8.4%
Older: 55+	26.0%	26.9%	22.8%	22.1%	15.2%

on the basis of their actual survey responses. The next column (labeled "Aggregated Probabilities: Respondents") aggregates the probability of the respondents falling into each of the demographic categories across all respondents (these are the probabilities that were used in weighting and do not account for the survey responses). These first two columns should, in theory, give similar values. The next two columns give the aggregated probabilities when summed across all surveyed veterans and then across the entire sample frame. Differences between the second column and the third and fourth columns indicate that the likelihood of response differs across the respective category. The final column gives our estimate as to the within-category response rates based upon an optimization algorithm, as described above. We see evidence that Black and Hispanic veterans are less likely to respond, and we see further evidence that younger veterans are less likely to respond.

Survey Measures

The survey gathered information about the health and well-being of veterans in New York. We asked about physical and mental health needs and service use. We also asked about other types of services veterans in New York were using or would like to use. In general, the health and well-being questions and scales were chosen to match those used in the 2010 study of veterans in New York (Farmer et al., 2011). Health care service use questions were expanded to explore differences in use and perceptions of care provided by VA and community providers.

Demographics and Military Experience

Survey respondents provided information on their age, gender, race/ethnicity, marital status, education level, employment status, and household income. They also provided information on their military experience, including years of service, highest rank achieved, branch of service, number of deployments to serve in a combat operation, and discharge status.

Health and Well-Being

Probable depression. Following the prior survey, we used the Patient Health Questionnaire (PHQ) to assess symptoms of major depression in veteran respondents (Farmer et al., 2011; Kroenke, Spitzer, and Williams, 2001, 2003; Kroenke et al., 2009). We use the PHQ-2, a screening variant of the PHQ-9, that asks about how often the respondent has been bothered by "little interest or pleasure in doing things" and "feeling down, depressed, and hopeless" (Kroenke, Spitzer, and Williams, 2003). We changed the duration for symptom reporting from two weeks to a month to coincide with the duration used for assessment of PTSD symptoms. Responses were provided on a four-point scale (0–3) ranging from "not at all" (0) to "nearly every day" (3). A respondent is identified as likely to have major depression if they receive a score of three or greater across these two items. We expect that by expanding the duration used for symptom reporting from two to four weeks, our estimate of probable depression is conservative as it may be less likely that someone experiences symptoms nearly every day over the longer reporting period.

Probable PTSD. To be consistent with the prior survey, we used the PTSD Checklist—Military Version (PCL-M) to assess probable PTSD (Weathers et al., 1994). The instrument contains 17 symptom items related to combat stress (e.g., repeated disturbing memories and dreams, feeling irritated or having angry outbursts, feeling jumpy or easily startled) that are based on the *DSM-IV*. An updated PTSD Checklist (PCL-5) based on revised diagnostic criteria in the *DSM-V* is available that includes three additional items and rewords many of the prior items (Blevins et al., 2015). While the two instruments are different, a growing body of evidence suggests that the two scales are comparable for epidemiological purposes, yielding similar prevalence estimates (Hoge et al., 2014; LeardMann et al., 2021). Responses to the symptom items were reported over the past four weeks on a five-point scale (0–4) reflecting how much the respondent has been bothered by each of the symptoms, ranging from "not at all" (0) to "extremely" (4). For scoring purposes, symptoms were counted as present if the respondent reported being at least "moderately" (3) bothered by the symptom. The symptoms were then scored based on *DSM-IV* to identify a probable PTSD diagnosis.

Suicide. To assess suicidal thoughts and behaviors, we used a set of three questions about thinking about, planning to, or attempting suicide. Specifically, respondents were asked whether over the past year they had seriously thought about trying to kill themselves. If the respondent answered this question affirmatively, they were asked whether they had made any plans to kill themselves and whether they had tried to kill themselves. These are the same questions used to assess suicidal thoughts and behaviors in the National Survey of Drug Use and Health (Substance Abuse and Mental Health Services Administration, 2023). After these questions were asked, respondents were provided with information about the National Suicide Prevention Lifeline and other resources. In addition, we asked all respondents whether they knew a veteran who had died by suicide.

Access to firearms. To assess firearm safety, we used the questions from the Behavioral Risk Factor Surveillance System (Centers for Disease Control and Prevention, 2023). We asked respondents whether firearms were kept in or around their house. If so, respondents were asked whether those firearms were loaded. If the firearms were loaded, respondents were asked whether they were stored in a way that required a key or combination to access them.

Physical health. Following the prior study, we assessed physical health using the Physical Functioning and Role Limitations Due to Physical Health subscales of the SF-36 (Ware et al., 1993). The Physical Functioning subscale is based on answers to questions about how much their health limits them in ten different activities (e.g., vigorous activities such as running, moderate activities such as playing golf, climbing one flight of stairs, bathing or dressing yourself). The Role Limitations Due to Physical Health subscale includes four items asking whether the respondent has problems with various work or other regular activities due to their physical health. The problems include cutting down time spent on work, accomplishing less than you would like, being limited in the kind of work you could do, and having difficulty performing your regular work or activities. Subscales are scored from 0 to 100, with higher scores indicating better physical health. The SF-36 and its subscales have been found to be valid and reliable measures of physical health (Brazier et al., 1992; Buchwald et al., 1996; Stansfeld, Roberts, and Foot, 1997; Ware et al., 1993). For purposes of comparison with the general population, we use the distribution of age and gender in our sample to adjust population mean scores from Ware et al. (1993). We also asked respondents to self-report their health status on a five-point scale ("poor," "fair," "good," "very good," or "excellent").

Disability status. To assess disability status, we asked respondents whether they had ever been rated as disabled or partially disabled by the either the military or VA. If so, they were asked to report their most recent disability rating (0–100 percent).

Exposure to toxic chemicals. Exposure to toxic chemicals during military service is an emerging issue we wanted to explore with veterans. We asked them whether they had any health conditions that they believed are related to exposure to toxic chemicals during their military service.

Alcohol and drug use. We assessed alcohol use during the past month by asking about the number of days on which respondents consumed alcohol and the number of days on which respondents engaged in binge drinking during the past 30 days. Binge drinking was defined as four or more drinks on one occasion for females and as five or more drinks on one occasion for males.

We assessed veterans' use of illicit substances over the past 12 months. We asked one question about illegal drugs, including cocaine, heroin, amphetamines, or ecstasy, and two questions about misuse of prescription medications (i.e., use of a medication that was not prescribed for the respondent by a doctor or was used in a way other than as prescribed). We also asked about past-year use of marijuana or cannabis products, which is legal for adults 21 and older in New York (see NYC Health, undated).

Food insecurity. We used the two-item Hunger Vital Sign to assess food insecurity among respondents (Hager et al., 2010). The look-back period is 12 months, and the questions ask about worrying about or experiencing a situation where their food would run out before they got money to buy more. A respondent is determined to be at risk for food insecurity if they answer "Yes" to either or both questions. The Hunger Vital Sign has been found to accurately identify adults at high risk of food insecurity (Gundersen et al., 2017).

Access to and Experience with Health Care Services

Access to health care. To assess access, we asked veterans to report their health insurance status (both having any and, if so, what type) and whether they had a usual source of health care.

Unmet need for care. To assess unmet need for care, we asked veterans whether there was any time in the last 12 months when they needed medical care but did not get it. If they reported having an unmet need, we asked about the potential barriers to care, including cost, inconvenient location or hours, lack of information about how to access services, and a lack of support services to facilitate receiving care (e.g., no transportation, no child care). Respondents could report multiple barriers.

We asked a similar set of questions to assess unmet need for mental health care. Among those that reported an unmet need for mental health care (i.e., needing mental health care in the last 12 months but not receiving it), we asked about potential barriers to care. In addition to the barriers considered for medical care, for mental health care we also included barriers related to the perceived effectiveness of care, stigma associated with care, and concerns about side effects of psychiatric medications.

Experience with VA health care. We were particularly interested in the experiences of veterans who have used VA health care services in the past year. We asked whether veterans had used health care services at a VA facility and whether they had used health care services from a community provider that were paid for by VA.

Among those that had received health care services at a VA facility, we asked about their experience and satisfaction with that care. The questions were adapted from the 2022 Survey of Veteran Enrollees' Health Use and Health Care (VA, 2022) and focused on the ease and convenience of accessing services (e.g., convenient hours, convenient location, ability to get specialist care) and their experience with the staff and medical providers, (e.g., shown respect, clear communication about options and choices, included in decisionmaking, privacy respected). We also asked about whether the health care provider they saw most often at the VA facility understood military culture and the health challenges facing veterans.

Among veterans who had received services from a community provider that were paid for by VA, we asked the same set of questions about their experiences and satisfaction with the services they received.

All respondents were asked about their preferences for where to receive health care: in a military treatment facility, in a VA facility, from a civilian provider not associated with the military or VA, or a civilian provider that you were referred to by VA. For those that reported a preference for care from a civilian provider, we asked them about their reasons for that preference. The possible reasons included that they had access to better care in the community, they already have a civilian provider they trust, they prefer to go to the same doctor as their spouse, they had easier and better access to civilian providers, they had a bad experience with VA in the past, they were not sure if they were eligible for VA services, and they did not know how to access VA services. Respondents were allowed to select all reasons that applied to them.

Use of Other Services for Veterans

Utilization, perceived helpfulness, and understanding of veterans' benefits and services. Respondents were asked about eight benefits and services available to them and whether they had used those benefits and services since leaving the military. We also asked which of these benefits and services they would consider helpful, regardless of whether they had used them. Finally, we asked whether they considered themselves to have a "good" understanding of the benefits available to veterans and knew how to get answers to questions about benefits.

Abbreviations

AAPOR	American Association of Public Opinion Research
CI	confidence interval
COVID-19	coronavirus disease 2019
CPS	Current Population Survey
DSM-IV	*Diagnostic and Statistical Manual of Mental Disorders, Fourth Edition*
LL	lower limit
MSA	metropolitan statistical area
NYS	New York State
OEF	Operation Enduring Freedom
OIF	Operation Iraqi Freedom
PACT Act	Sergeant First Class Heath Robinson Honoring Our Promise to Address Comprehensive Toxics Act of 2022
PCL-M	Posttraumatic Stress Disorder Checklist, adapted for military population
PHQ-2	Patient Health Questionnaire, 2-item measure
PTSD	posttraumatic stress disorder
RONA	request for names and addresses
SF-36	36-Item Short Form Health Survey
SNAP	Supplemental Nutrition Assistance Program
UL	upper limit
USPS	United States Postal Service
VA	Department of Veterans Affairs
VHA	Veterans Health Administration

References

AAPOR—*See* American Association of Public Opinion Research.

Agency for Healthcare Research and Quality, "MEPS Household Component: Accessibility and Quality of Care: Access to Care," webpage, 2021. As of June 24, 2024:
https://datatools.ahrq.gov/meps-hc/?tab=accessibility-and-quality-of-care&dash=14

American Association of Public Opinion Research, "Response Rates Calculator," webpage, undated. As of July 9, 2024:
https://aapor.org/response-rates/

Benson, C., *Poverty in States and Metropolitan Areas: 2022*, ACSBR-016, U.S. Census Bureau, December 4, 2023.

Bernard, D. M., and T. M. Selden, "Access to Care Among Nonelderly Veterans," *Medical Care*, Vol. 54, No. 3, 2016.

Betancourt, J. A., D. M. Dolezel, R. Shanmugam, G. J. Pacheco, P. Stigler Granados, and L. V. Fulton, "The Health Status of the US Veterans: A Longitudinal Analysis of Surveillance Data Prior to and During the COVID-19 Pandemic," *Healthcare*, Vol. 11, No. 14, 2023.

Blevins, C. A., F. W. Weathers, M. T. Davis, T. K. Witte, and J. L. Domino, "The Posttraumatic Stress Disorder Checklist for DSM-5 (PCL-5): Development and Initial Psychometric Evaluation," *Journal of Traumatic Stress*, Vol. 28, No. 6, 2015.

Brazier, J. E., R. Harper, N. Jones, A. O'Cathain, K. J. Thomas, T. Usherwood, and L. Westlake, "Validating the SF-36 Health Survey Questionnaire: New Outcome Measure for Primary Care," *British Medical Journal*, Vol. 305, No. 6846, 1992.

Brostow, D. P., E. Gunzburger, and K. S. Thomas, "Food Insecurity Among Veterans: Findings from the Health and Retirement Study," *Journal of Nutrition, Health & Aging*, Vol. 21, No. 10, 2017.

Buchwald, D., T. Pearlman, J. Umali, K. Schmaling, and W. Katon, "Functional Status in Patients with Chronic Fatigue Syndrome, Other Fatiguing Illnesses, and Healthy Individuals," *American Journal of Medicine*, Vol. 101, No. 4, 1996.

Centers for Disease Control and Prevention, *Behavioral Risk Factor Surveillance System Survey Questionnaire*, U.S. Department of Health and Human Services, August 29, 2023.

Chari, Ramya, Heather M. Salazar, and Lauren Skrabala, *Lessons from 9/11 for Supporting Veterans Exposed to Military Environmental Hazards: Veterans' Issues in Focus*, RAND Corporation, PE-A1363-11, 2024. As of August 19, 2024:
https://www.rand.org/pubs/perspectives/PEA1363-11.html

Cohen, J., *Statistical Power Analysis for the Behavioral Sciences*, Routledge, 2013.

Cohen, R. A., and P. Boersma, "Financial Burden of Medical Care Among Veterans Aged 25–64, by Health Insurance Coverage: United States, 2019–2021," *National Health Statistics Reports*, No. 182, March 2023.

Department of Veterans Affairs, *2022 Survey of Veteran Enrollees' Health and Use of Health Care Findings Report*, December 2022.

Department of Veterans Affairs, *2023 National Veteran Suicide Prevention Annual Report*, 2023.

Department of Veterans Affairs, *Statistical Trends: Veterans with a Service-Connected Disability, 1990 to 2018*, May 2019.

Department of Veterans Affairs, *VA PACT Act Performance Dashboard*, No. 37, July 5, 2024.

Dubowitz, Tamara, *Food Insecurity Among Veterans: Veterans' Issues in Focus*, RAND Corporation, PE-A1363-2, 2021. As of August 19, 2024:
https://www.rand.org/pubs/perspectives/PEA1363-2.html

Dubowitz, Tamara, Andrea S. Richardson, Teague Ruder, and Catria Gadwah-Meaden, *Reducing Policy Barriers to SNAP Participation by Food-Insecure Veterans*, RAND Corporation, RB-A1363-1, 2023. As of August 19, 2024:
https://www.rand.org/pubs/research_briefs/RBA1363-1.html

Elliott, M. N., P. A. Morrison, A. Fremont, D. F. McCaffrey, P. Pantoja, and N. Lurie, "Using the Census Bureau's Surname List to Improve Estimates of Race/Ethnicity and Associated Disparities," *Health Services and Outcomes Research Methodology*, Vol. 9, No. 2, 2009.

Farmer, Carrie M., Lisa H. Jaycox, Grant N. Marshall, Terry L. Schell, Terri Tanielian, Christine Anne Vaughan, and Glenda Wrenn, *A Needs Assessment of New York State Veterans: Final Report to the New York State Health Foundation*, RAND Corporation, TR-920-NYSHF, 2011. As of August 19, 2024:
https://www.rand.org/pubs/technical_reports/TR920.html

Friar, N. W., F. Merrill-Francis, E. M. Parker, C. Siordia, and T. R. Simon, "Firearm Storage Behaviors—Behavioral Risk Factor Surveillance System, Eight States, 2021–2022," *Morbidity and Mortality Weekly Report*, Vol. 73, No. 23, 2024.

Goldstein, R. B., S. M. Smith, S. P. Chou, T. D. Saha, J. Jung, H. Zhang, R. P. Pickering, W. J. Ruan, B. Huang, and B. F. Grant, "The Epidemiology of DSM-5 Posttraumatic Stress Disorder in the United States: Results from the National Epidemiologic Survey on Alcohol and Related Conditions-III," *Social Psychiatry and Psychiatric Epidemiology*, Vol. 51, 2016.

Goodwin, R. D., L. C. Dierker, M. Wu, S. Galea, C. W. Hoven, and A. H. Weinberger, "Trends in US Depression Prevalence from 2015 to 2020: The Widening Treatment Gap," *American Journal of Preventive Medicine*, Vol. 63, No. 5, 2022.

Grogan, N., E. Moore, B. Peabody, M. Seymour, and K. M. Williams, *New York State Minority Veteran Needs Assessment*, Center for a New American Security, February 2020.

Gundersen, C., E. E. Engelhard, A. S. Crumbaugh, and H. K. Seligman, "Brief Assessment of Food Insecurity Accurately Identifies High-Risk US Adults," *Public Health Nutrition*, Vol. 20, No. 8, 2017.

Hager, E. R., A. M. Quigg, M. M. Black, S. M. Coleman, T. Heeren, R. Rose-Jacobs, J. T. Cook, S. A. E. de Cuba, P. H. Casey, and M. Chilton, "Development and Validity of a 2-Item Screen to Identify Families at Risk for Food Insecurity," *Pediatrics*, Vol. 126, No. 1, 2010.

Hoge, C. W., L. A. Riviere, J. E. Wilk, R. K. Herrell, and F. W. Weathers, "The Prevalence of Post-Traumatic Stress Disorder (PTSD) in US Combat Soldiers: A Head-to-Head Comparison of DSM-5 Versus DSM-IV-TR Symptom Criteria with the PTSD Checklist," *Lancet Psychiatry*, Vol. 1, No. 4, 2014.

Institute of Medicine, *Returning Home from Iraq and Afghanistan: Preliminary Assessment of Readjustment Needs of Veterans, Service Members, and Their Families*, National Academies Press, 2010.

IPUMS CPS, "Veterans Supplement Sample Notes," webpage, undated. As of August 22, 2024:
https://cps.ipums.org/cps/vet_sample_notes.shtml

Ivey-Stephenson, A. Z., A. E. Crosby, J. M. Hoenig, S. Gyawali, E. Park-Lee, and S. L. Hedden, "Suicidal Thoughts and Behaviors Among Adults Aged ≥18 Years—United States, 2015–2019," *Morbidity and Mortality Weekly Report Surveillance Summaries*, Vol. 71, No. 1, 2022.

Kroenke, K., R. L. Spitzer, and J. B. W. Williams, "The Patient Health Questionnaire-2: Validity of a Two-Item Depression Screener," *Medical Care*, Vol. 41, No. 11, 2003.

Kroenke, K., R. L. Spitzer, and J. B. W. Williams, "The PHQ-9: Validity of a Brief Depression Severity Measure," *Journal of General Internal Medicine*, Vol. 16, No. 9, 2001.

Kroenke, K., T. W. Strine, R. L. Spitzer, J. B. W. Williams, J. T. Berry, and A. H. Mokdad, "The PHQ-8 as a Measure of Current Depression in the General Population," *Journal of Affective Disorders*, Vol. 114, No. 1, 2009.

LeardMann, C. A., H. S. McMaster, S. Warner, A. P. Esquivel, B. Porter, T. M. Powell, X. M. Tu, W. W. Lee, R.P. Rull, and C. W. Hoge, "Comparison of Posttraumatic Stress Disorder Checklist Instruments from *Diagnostic and Statistical Manual of Mental Disorders, Fourth Edition* vs *Fifth Edition* in a Large Cohort of US Military Service Members and Veterans," *JAMA Network Open*, Vol. 4, No. 4, 2021.

Li, S., S. Huang, S. Hu, and J. Lai, "Psychological Consequences Among Veterans During the COVID-19 Pandemic: A Scoping Review," *Psychiatry Research*, Vol. 324, 2023.

London, A. S., and C. M. Heflin, "Supplemental Nutrition Assistance Program (SNAP) Use Among Active-Duty Military Personnel, Veterans, and Reservists," *Population Research and Policy Review*, Vol. 34, No. 6, 2015.

Moradi, Y., B. Dowran, and M. Sepandi, "The Global Prevalence of Depression, Suicide Ideation, and Attempts in the Military Forces: A Systematic Review and Meta-Analysis of Cross Sectional Studies," *BMC Psychiatry*, Vol. 21, 2021.

Na, P. J., P. P. Schnurr, and R. H. Pietrzak, "Mental Health of US Combat Veterans by War Era: Results from the National Health and Resilience in Veterans Study," *Journal of Psychiatric Research*, Vol. 158, 2023.

National Center for Health Statistics, *Health, United States, 2020–2021: Table HStat: Respondent-Assessed Fair-Poor Health Status, by Selected Characteristics: United States, Selected Years 1991–2019*, 2023. As of August 22, 2024:
https://www.cdc.gov/nchs/data/hus/2020-2021/HStat.pdf

New York State Department of Health, "Veterans Health Information Clearing House," webpage, July 2023. As of August 22, 2024:
https://www.health.ny.gov/health_care/veterans/

New York State Senate, "Consolidated Laws of New York, Chapter 13: Veterans' Services, Article 1, Section 25," webpage, October 6, 2023. As of August 22, 2024:
https://www.nysenate.gov/legislation/laws/VET/25

NYC Health, "Cannabis (Marijuana)," webpage, undated. As of June 20, 2024:
https://www.nyc.gov/site/doh/health/health-topics/marijuana.page#:~:text=Legal%20Adult%20Use%20and%20Possession,laws%2C%20with%20a%20few%20exceptions

NYS Office of Information Technology Services, NYS Veterans, mobile application, July 31, 2024.

Office of the Assistant Secretary for Planning and Evaluation, "Poverty Guidelines," webpage, January 17, 2024. As of June 14, 2024:
https://aspe.hhs.gov/topics/poverty-economic-mobility/poverty-guidelines

Parast, L., M. Mathews, M. Elliott, A. Tolpadi, E. Flow-Delwiche, W. G. Lehrman, D. Stark, and K. Becker, "Effects of Push-to-Web Mixed Mode Approaches on Survey Response Rates: Evidence from a Randomized Experiment in Emergency Departments," *Survey Practice*, Vol. 12, No. 1, 2019.

Patrick, M. E., R. A. Miech, L. D. Johnston, and P. M. O'Malley, *Monitoring the Future Panel Study Annual Report: National Data on Substance Use Among Adults Ages 19 to 60, 1976–2022*, Institute for Social Research, 2023.

Peterson-KFF Health System Tracker, "Usual Source of Care," webpage, 2022. As of June 24, 2024: https://www.healthsystemtracker.org/indicator/access-affordability/usual-source-care/#Percent%20of%20adults%20who%20reported%20not%20having%20a%20usual%20source%20of%20care,%202008-2022

Public Law 113-146, Veterans' Access to Care Through Choice, Accountability, and Transparency Act of 2014, August 7, 2014.

Public Law 115-182, John S. McCain III, Daniel K. Akaka, and Samuel R. Johnson VA Maintaining Internal Systems and Strengthening Integrated Outside Networks Act of 2018, June 6, 2018.

Public Law 116-117, Commander John Scott Hannon Veterans Mental Health Care Improvement Act of 2020, October 17, 2020.

Public Law 117-168, Sergeant First Class Heath Robinson Honoring Our Promise to Address Comprehensive Toxics Act of 2022, August 10, 2022.

Rabbitt, M. P., L. J. Hales, M. P. Burke, and A. Coleman-Jensen, *Household Food Security in the United States in 2022*, Economic Research Service, U.S. Department of Agriculture, October 2023.

Rabbitt, M. P., and M. D. Smith, *Food Insecurity Among Working-Age Veterans*, Economic Research Service, U.S. Department of Agriculture, May 2021.

Ramchand, Rajeev, *Suicide Among Veterans: Veterans' Issues in Focus*, RAND Corporation, PE-A1363-1, 2021. As of August 19, 2024: https://www.rand.org/pubs/perspectives/PEA1363-1.html

Robinson, Eric, Justin W. Lee, Teague Ruder, Megan S. Schuler, Gilad Wenig, Carrie M. Farmer, Jessica Phillips, and Rajeev Ramchand, *A Summary of Veteran-Related Statistics*, RAND Corporation, RR-A1363-5, 2023. As of August 19, 2024: https://www.rand.org/pubs/research_reports/RRA1363-5.html

Sauermann, H., and M. Roach, "Increasing Web Survey Response Rates in Innovation Research: An Experimental Study of Static and Dynamic Contact Design Features," *Research Policy*, Vol. 42, No. 1, 2013.

Schnittker, J., "Scars: The Long-term Effects of Combat Exposure on Health," *Socius*, Vol. 4, 2018.

Simonetti, J. A., D. Azrael, A. Rowhani-Rahbar, and M. Miller, "Firearm Storage Practices Among American Veterans," *American Journal of Preventive Medicine*, Vol. 55, No. 4, 2018.

Stansfeld, S. A., R. Roberts, and S. Foot, "Assessing the Validity of the SF-36 General Health Survey," *Quality of Life Research*, Vol. 6, No. 3, 1997.

Substance Abuse and Mental Health Services Administration, *2022 National Survey on Drug Use and Health (NSDUH): Methodological Summary and Definitions*, November 2023.

Tanielian, Terri, Lisa H. Jaycox, Terry L. Schell, Grant N. Marshall, M. Audrey Burnam, Christine Eibner, Benjamin R. Karney, Lisa S. Meredith, Jeanne S. Ringel, and Mary E. Vaiana, *Invisible Wounds of War: Summary and Recommendations for Addressing Psychological and Cognitive Injuries*, RAND Corporation, MS-720/1-CCF, 2008. As of August 19, 2024: https://www.rand.org/pubs/monographs/MG720z1.html

Teplova, A. E., H. A. H. M. Bakker, S. I. B., Perry, F. S. Van Etten-Jamaludin, M.-C. J. Plat, and M. B. M. Bekkers, "The Impact of Deployment and Combat Exposure on Physical Health Among Military Personnel: A Systematic Review of Incidence, Prevalence, and Risks," *Military Medicine*, Vol. 187, Nos. 9–10, 2022.

Twenge, J. M., A. B. Cooper, T. E. Joiner, M. E. Duffy, and S. G. Binau, "Age, Period, and Cohort Trends in Mood Disorder Indicators and Suicide-Related Outcomes in a Nationally Representative Dataset, 2005–2017," *Journal of Abnormal Psychology*, Vol. 128, No. 3, 2019.

VA—*See* Department of Veterans Affairs.

Vespa, J., *Aging Veterans: America's Veteran Population in Later Life*, ACS-54, U.S. Census Bureau, July 2023.

Villarroel, M. A., and E. P. Terlizzi, *Symptoms of Depression Among Adults: United States, 2019*, National Center for Health Statistics, 2020.

Ware, J. E., K. K. Snow, M. Kosinski, and B. Gandek, *SF-36 Health Survey: Manual and Interpretation Guide*, Health Institute, New England Medical Center, 1993.

Weathers, F., B. Litz, J. Huska, and T. Keane, *PTSD Checklist—Military Version*, Behavioral Science Division, National Center for PTSD, 1994.

Widome, R., A. Jensen, A. Bangerter, and S. S. Fu, "Food Insecurity Among Veterans of the US Wars in Iraq and Afghanistan," *Public Health Nutrition*, Vol. 18, No. 5, 2015.